DADS IN THE FOURTH TRIMESTER

What Every Husband Needs to Know About

Life After Baby

Marc Seffelaar

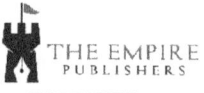

THE EMPIRE
PUBLISHERS

12808 West Airport Blvd Suite 270M Sugar Land, TX
77478, Unites States

https://www.theempirepublishers.com/

Our books may be purchased in bulk for promotional, educational, or business use.

Please contact The Empire Publishers at +1 844 636-4579, or by email at support@theempirepublishers.com

First Edition December 2025

About the author

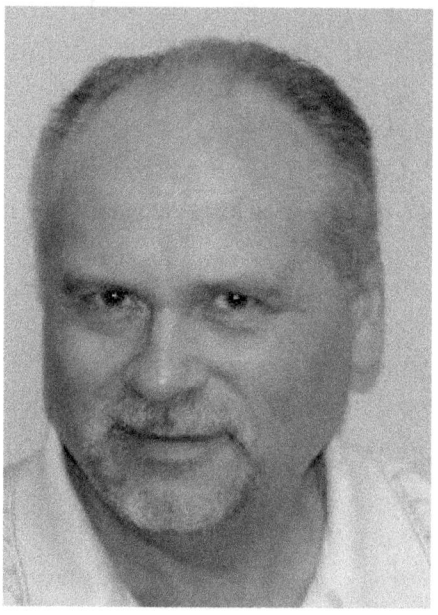

Marc Seffelaar is a Saskatchewan-born author with over 38 years of experience in accounting, financial planning, and business consulting. A survivor of a life-altering accident in 1995, and more than 30 surgeries, Marc's journey through trauma, addiction, and ultimately spiritual recovery fuels the deeply personal, grace-filled perspective behind his writing.

Marc holds a Bachelor of Commerce, an MBA, a PhD, and several professional certifications. His books combine practical wisdom with emotional and spiritual depth, offering clear guidance for life's most challenging seasons, from estate planning and emotional wellness to recovery from addiction and daily self-compassion.

He is the author of Be Kind to Yourself, Legacy Unlocked, and several other titles that support readers in reclaiming peace, purpose, and clarity. Marc also partners with Dr. Lindy Summers to co-author meaningful resources for new and expectant mothers, blending faith, health, and emotional support for one of life's most sacred transitions.

Marc writes for everyday people looking for honest answers, spiritual renewal, and the courage to begin again, one peaceful, grace-filled step at a time.

Dedication

To the dads who stayed, showed up, and figured it out one sleepless night at a time, this is for you.

To the men quietly holding the weight of new beginnings, who may not always have the words but offer their presence, you are seen.

To my own children, you've taught me more about fatherhood than any book ever could.

And to the moms who trust us, love us, and let us learn beside them, thank you.

—Marc Seffelaar, PhD

Acknowledgments

This book would not exist without the love, wisdom, and support of many people whose kindness shaped every page.

To my family, especially my wife and children, thank you for walking this journey with me. Your patience, prayers, and laughter sustained me on the hard days and celebrated with me on the good ones. You are my reason and my reward.

To my editor and publishing team, thank you for believing in this message and sharpening my words with care and excellence. You helped me say what I meant clearly, beautifully, and truthfully.

To Dr. Lindy Summers, thank you for lending your clinical experience, insight, and heart to this book. Your years of walking with new moms brought a depth of compassion that makes this work stronger and more relevant.

To the early readers, mentors, and friends who reviewed drafts, offered thoughtful feedback, and spoke encouragement over this project, your voices helped me stay the course. I am deeply grateful.

To The Empire Publishers, thank you for your professionalism, your passion for meaningful books, and your continued support of this vision.

And above all, I thank God, for the grace to keep going, the strength to be honest, and the healing that made it possible to turn pain into purpose.

This is not just my book, it belongs to every person who helped carry it.

With deepest thanks,

Marc Seffelaar, PhD

Table of Contents

Introduction...1

Chapter 1: Embracing the New Role...............................5

Chapter 2: Connecting with Your Newborn.....................21

Chapter 3: Supporting Your Partner.............................34

Chapter 4: Handling the Home Front 48

Chapter 5: Maintaining Mental Wellness.......................63

Chapter 6: Navigating Work-Life Balance 74

Chapter 7: Understanding Baby Development...............84

Chapter 8: Overcoming Challenges Together 95

Chapter 9: Building a Strong Parenting Partnership.....105

Chapter 10: Embracing Change and Growth...............115

Chapter 11 Cultivating Community and Connection 125

Chapter 12: Looking Forward – The Long-Term Dad.....136

Introduction

It was 3:00 a.m. The baby had been crying for what felt like an eternity, her tiny voice piercing through the stillness of the night. I stood alone in the soft glow of the nursery, gently rocking her in my arms, every muscle in my body aching from exhaustion. My eyes were heavy, my patience wearing thin. I could hear the faint hum of the white noise machine and the soft creaks of the wooden floor beneath my tired feet. My wife was finally asleep in the next room, stealing a few precious hours of rest she so desperately needed.

In that quiet, sleepless hour, something shifted in me. I understood, perhaps for the first time, that fatherhood wasn't just about being physically present, it was about showing up in the moments that tested me the most. It was about being steady when everything felt chaotic. Being a dad meant choosing involvement over distance, patience over frustration, and compassion over confusion.

This book, *Dads in the Fourth Trimester: What Every Husband Needs to Know About Life After Baby*, was born from those raw, bewildering nights. It came out of the desperate searches I made at 4 a.m., looking for guidance and finding page after page aimed at mothers. There were hundreds of books on motherhood, yet almost none that spoke directly to the man holding the crying baby, wondering if he was doing anything right. I wrote this to fill that void: a real, honest guide for dads who want to be more than bystanders in those first chaotic months of life after birth.

My vision is straightforward: to create a practical, no-fluff handbook for new fathers, something rooted in emotional truth and everyday reality. This book is for men ready to step into fatherhood with open eyes and willing hands. It's about understanding your partner's changing emotional landscape, learning to connect with your baby, and figuring out how to care for yourself so you don't get lost in the process.

Let's be honest, new dads are thrown into the deep end. There are endless sleepless nights, the pressure to "be strong" for your partner, the sheer confusion of handling a newborn who can't communicate anything clearly. These moments are shared by fathers everywhere, yet we rarely talk about them. This book is here to start that conversation. It offers tools, stories, and strategies to help you not only survive but grow through this transformation.

The inspiration behind this book is deeply personal. Becoming a father changed me in ways I couldn't have predicted. I watched my wife become a mother: her strength, her struggles, her vulnerability. I didn't always know what to say or do, and I made plenty of mistakes. But through it all, I learned. And now, years later, watching my own daughters become mothers has brought a whole new depth to my understanding. I've seen how essential fathers are, not just in the delivery room, but every single day after.

In the chapters ahead, we'll walk through key topics every new dad should know. We'll dive into emotional awareness, how to recognize the signs of postpartum anxiety or depression, how to be a sounding board and a steady hand. We'll get practical, too, from mastering the art of a midnight diaper change to making sure your partner has a glass of water before nursing. We'll also cover how to maintain your relationship, build trust, and make space for your own emotional needs without guilt or shame.

I've had the honor of co-authoring this book with Dr. Lindy Summers, a leading expert in postpartum health. Her voice brings essential clinical insight and research-backed advice, balanced with warmth and humanity. Our combined perspectives, one from lived experience, the other from professional expertise, make this book both deeply relatable and genuinely useful.

Each chapter is designed as a stepping stone through the fourth trimester. You'll learn what to expect, how to adapt, and how to thrive as a new dad. We want this book to be your companion, something you can return to in the middle of the night, dog-eared and coffee-stained, when you just need to know you're not alone.

So as you turn the pages, I invite you to reflect. Think about your own story. Be honest with yourself. Be gentle with your learning curve. And most importantly, stay connected: to your partner, your baby, and yourself.

By the end of this book, you'll have a clearer picture of what this season really demands, and what it can give you in return. You'll walk away not just more informed, but more confident, more grounded, and more emotionally available.

Welcome to the fourth trimester. It's messy. It's beautiful. It's real. And you're exactly where you need to be.

Let's begin.

Chapter 1:
Embracing the New Role

A few months ago, I found myself standing in the middle of a cluttered nursery, tools in one hand, a half-assembled crib in the other, wondering how my life had changed so completely, and so quickly. Just the night before, we were still two people waiting. Now, we were a family. My wife rested in her hospital bed down the hall, cradling our newborn in a haze of exhaustion and wonder. Meanwhile, I was elbow-deep in screws, instructions, and self-doubt, fumbling my way through my first act of fatherhood. In that quiet, chaotic moment, I realized that being a dad isn't about a title, it's about transformation. This chapter is your invitation to lean into that transformation and begin shaping not just your identity as a father, but as a fully present, emotionally engaged, and confident parent.

From Dude to Dad:
Becoming a father is a profound shift. An internal earthquake that shakes up your priorities, identity, and understanding of what it means to love someone more than you love yourself. It's not just about wearing the "dad" label; it's about stepping into an

entirely new role that redefines your sense of self.

This transformation doesn't happen all at once. At first, it may feel like you're simply playing a part, going through the motions while your inner compass recalibrates. You may grieve pieces of your old life: the spontaneous late-night hangouts, the undisturbed sleep, the solo time that once recharged you. That grief is real and valid. But in time, you'll begin to notice something else: a growing sense of purpose, a deepening emotional wellspring, and a newfound strength that emerges from showing up, even when you don't feel ready.

You are not losing yourself; you're expanding.

Who Are You Becoming?

One of the most powerful things you can do during this transition is to consciously craft your narrative of fatherhood. Who are you now? Who do you want to be for your child and your partner?

Start by creating your own fatherhood mission statement. This is your blueprint, your anchor when things feel overwhelming. Your mission statement doesn't have to be lofty or poetic. It just needs to be *real*. For instance:

- *"I want to be the kind of dad who listens without judgment."*
- *"I commit to being emotionally present and physically available."*
- *"I want my child to feel safe and unconditionally loved in my presence."*

Revisiting this statement during moments of self-doubt can ground you, reminding you why you're doing this, and who you're becoming in the process.

Keeping a Part of Yourself:
It's easy to feel like everything must be sacrificed at the altar of fatherhood. While sacrifices are inevitable, losing *yourself* entirely isn't sustainable or healthy. Your passions, hobbies, and personal time are not just "nice to have"—they're vital lifelines that make you more centered and emotionally available.

Whether it's taking 30 minutes to play the guitar, read, hit the gym, or simply sit in silence, carving out time for yourself doesn't mean you're neglecting your family. It means you're recharging so you can show up fully.

Celebrating Small Wins:
One of the fastest ways to grow as a new dad is to notice, and celebrate, the small victories. They may seem trivial, but they are powerful affirmations that you're learning and adapting. Whether it's successfully calming your baby at 3 a.m., making your partner a meal she didn't have to ask for, or surviving your first solo outing with the baby, *these moments matter.*

I still remember the first time I changed a diaper without a blowout or panic attack. I felt like I deserved a trophy. These are the invisible milestones of fatherhood. Give yourself credit. Every day that you show up counts.

Find Your Village:
Fatherhood can feel isolating, especially if you're trying to keep up a strong exterior. But connection is key. Talking to other dads, even virtually, can

normalize your experience and give you much-needed perspective. No one expects you to have all the answers, and sometimes hearing "me too" is all it takes to feel grounded.

Whether it's through local dad groups, parenting forums, or simply grabbing coffee with another new father, surround yourself with voices who understand the unique challenges and joys of this phase.

And don't hesitate to lean on family and friends. Accepting help isn't a sign of weakness; it's a recognition that parenting was never meant to be done alone.

Reflection Exercise:
Grab a journal or the notes app on your phone. Ask yourself:
- What kind of dad do I want to be?
- What values do I want to pass down?
- What moments do I hope my child remembers?
- Who has modeled great parenting for me, and what did I learn from them?

Use your answers to write a short mission statement. Let it be honest, aspirational, and something you can revisit often. This statement isn't set in stone, it will evolve as you do, but it offers clarity and intention during the foggy days of new parenthood.

Building Consistency in New Routines
Routines may not sound glamorous, but they're one of the most powerful tools in your fatherhood toolkit. Establishing rituals, like morning cuddles, bedtime stories, or Saturday morning walks, provides predictability for your child and a sense of stability for

you.

These routines become the rhythm of your new life, creating shared experiences that strengthen your bond and reduce stress. They're also part of what your child will remember. In a world that is constantly shifting, your consistency becomes their anchor.

Facing the Fear: Tackling Anxiety and Self-Doubt

Becoming a father can feel like stepping into unfamiliar territory with no map, no manual, and the pressure of getting everything "right" from the start. One moment, you're navigating your life with a sense of control, and the next, you're holding a tiny, fragile human whose entire world now revolves around you. It's no surprise that anxiety and self-doubt creep in, whispering questions like: *Am I cut out for this? What if I mess up? What if I'm not enough?*

These fears are more common than many new dads realize. And they're not a sign of weakness, they're a reflection of how deeply you care.

You're Not Alone

It's important to know that you're not the only one lying awake at 3 a.m., wondering if you're doing this right. Millions of new fathers experience similar doubts, about bonding with their baby, about being emotionally present, about whether they can provide the kind of stable, nurturing environment they desperately want to offer. These worries are rooted in love, not failure. And the moment you recognize and name your fears, you take away some of their power. What was once a vague sense of dread becomes something you can confront, unpack, and begin to manage.

Naming the Fears
Some of the most common fears include:
- **Not bonding with your baby**: Will they recognize you? Will you know how to comfort them?
- **Being a financial or emotional provider**: Can you carry the weight of responsibility without cracking?
- **Fear of making mistakes**: What if a misstep harms your child or damages their future?

These aren't irrational fears. They're rooted in the very real and profound responsibility of parenthood. But while the fear may be real, it doesn't have to dictate your experience.

Tools for Easing the Pressure
Managing anxiety starts with small, intentional steps. One of the simplest and most effective techniques is deep breathing. In moments when you feel overwhelmed, when the crying won't stop, when sleep deprivation hits hard, pause. Find a quiet space, even if it's the bathroom or the car. Close your eyes. Inhale slowly and deeply through your nose for four counts. Hold for four. Then exhale slowly through your mouth for four counts. Repeat this rhythm until you feel your heart rate slow and your thoughts become less chaotic. It only takes a minute, but the impact can be grounding.

Beyond breathing, **mindfulness** is another powerful practice. This doesn't require a meditation cushion or an hour of silence, just a few minutes of presence. Sit quietly, focus on your breath, and when thoughts rush in (they will), let them come and go without judgment. The goal isn't to control your thoughts, but to stop them from controlling you.

Mindfulness, over time, helps anchor you in the moment. It reminds you that you're doing the best you can *right now*, which is often exactly what your child needs.

When to Seek Help—and Why It's Okay

Sometimes, anxiety goes deeper than temporary stress. If you find yourself constantly on edge, struggling to sleep, or overwhelmed to the point that it interferes with daily life, it's time to consider speaking to a professional. Therapy isn't a last resort, it's a resource. It's a courageous step toward clarity, strength, and healing. In therapy, you can unpack old patterns, gain insight into the roots of your fears, and learn strategies that will benefit not just your parenting, but your overall mental health.

There is no shame in asking for help. In fact, doing so sets an incredible example for your child: that vulnerability is not weakness, and seeking support is a powerful, responsible choice.

Building Confidence One Win at a Time

Confidence as a dad doesn't come from knowing everything, it comes from showing up. From being willing to learn. From stacking small wins like bricks, building a foundation of trust in yourself.

Start a journal, not of perfect moments, but of real

ones. Write down what went well today. Maybe you got your baby to smile after a fussy hour. Maybe you figured out how to work the baby monitor. Maybe you remembered to pack the diaper bag without forgetting the wipes. These are victories. Celebrate them.

Set small, attainable goals. Don't aim to master everything at once. Focus on just one part of parenting, maybe you're in charge of bath time or morning feedings. As you get more comfortable, you can take on more. Each milestone boosts your belief that *yes, you can do this.*

Appreciating Your Unique Fatherhood Path

Every dad's journey is different. Some fall into a rhythm quickly. Others take longer to find their footing. There's no single "right" way to be a father, no universal timeline for feeling competent or confident. Avoid the trap of comparison. Instead, focus on your growth. Appreciate how you are showing up, how you are evolving, and how each day adds a new layer to your experience.

Reflect on the kind of father *you* want to be, not the one social media glorifies or pop culture stereotypes. Your path is yours to shape. And it will be shaped not by perfection, but by effort, presence, and love.

Redefining Masculinity in Fatherhood

Masculinity, as defined by previous generations, often came with rigid rules and a narrow blueprint. Strength was equated with silence, leadership with dominance, and love with provision. The ideal man was stoic, composed, and emotionally armored. But as we evolve in our roles as fathers, partners, and men, it becomes clear: these outdated ideals no longer serve us, or our families.

Stepping into fatherhood is not just about changing diapers or providing financial support; it's a profound opportunity to redefine what it means to be a man. It's a moment when the outdated armor of traditional masculinity begins to crack, revealing something far more authentic underneath: emotional depth, vulnerability, empathy, and connection. The world may still whisper that men should "man up" or "keep it together," but the truth is, real strength lies in the courage to show up fully, not just as providers or protectors, but as nurturers and listeners.

Many of us were raised by fathers who were emotionally distant, not because they didn't love us, but because they were taught to express love in limited, often material ways. They carried burdens they never named, fears they never voiced. Now, we stand at a crossroads: Do we repeat those patterns, or do we choose something better?

Redefining masculinity in the context of fatherhood means embracing a wider emotional spectrum. It means recognizing that being present for your child is not just about attending the soccer game or fixing a broken toy, it's about kneeling down, looking them in the eyes, and saying, "I understand." It's about admitting when you're scared, when you've made a mistake, and when you're unsure. Vulnerability, once framed as weakness, is now a superpower.

Imagine sitting beside your child after a rough day and telling them about a time you struggled too. That moment becomes more than a story, it becomes a bridge. Vulnerability teaches your child that it's okay to feel, to stumble, and to try again. It's a lesson far more valuable than any lecture about toughness or endurance.

Likewise, sharing your fears with your partner builds intimacy. Saying "I'm overwhelmed" doesn't make you less of a man, it makes you more human, more connected. You model emotional bravery, and in doing so, you give your family permission to do the same.

Embracing Emotional Expression

Love is not just something you feel, it's something you show. Affection isn't confined to birthday hugs or obligatory "I love yous." It's built into the way you listen without interrupting, the way you comfort your child without fixing their feelings, and the way you support your partner even when you're running on empty.

Children internalize what they see. When they witness a father who expresses love openly, they grow up believing that emotions are not gendered, they are human. When they see their father cry, apologize, or celebrate with unfiltered joy, they learn that emotional fluency is not only acceptable but essential.

Modeling a New Masculinity

Fatherhood gives you the chance to embody an inclusive, cooperative, and emotionally intelligent masculinity. It's reflected in how you co-parent, how you manage conflict, and how you participate in the day-to-day rhythms of family life. Washing dishes, packing lunches, or staying home with a sick child aren't signs of emasculation, they are signs of presence. And presence is power.

Let your children see your partnership thrive on teamwork rather than tradition. Let them see mutual respect in action, not just in words, but in chores, decisions, and compromises. Teach them through your actions that masculinity includes patience, flexibility, and emotional labor.

Invite them into conversations about values, about kindness, justice, and respect. These discussions are more than just words; they are seeds that grow into the ethics your children carry with them into the world.

Crafting a Legacy

Redefining masculinity isn't just about improving your present, it's about shaping the future. Your child will grow up remembering how you made them feel safe, heard, and cherished. They'll recall the nights you stayed up with them, not just to rock them back to sleep, but to soothe their fears with your presence. Start building your legacy with intention. Volunteer. Mentor. Share your story with other dads. Your vulnerability might be the exact thing another father needs to hear. Storytelling is healing. It connects us to one another and gives shape to the emotional terrain we often wander alone.

Case Study: The Strength of Opening Up

Consider the story of Kevin, a father who felt paralyzed with guilt after yelling at his toddler during a moment of exhaustion. Ashamed and overwhelmed, he opened up to another dad at the playground. To his surprise, the other father nodded in understanding and shared a similar experience. That conversation didn't erase Kevin's guilt, but it transformed it. He began to see himself not as a failure, but as a man learning in real time. That shift made space for growth, and compassion.

Role Reversal and Shared Strength

In many modern homes, traditional gender roles are being reshaped. Maybe your partner is the breadwinner, while you take on the bulk of the caregiving. Maybe you're both balancing careers and parenting, sharing roles without a script. These shifts are not threats to masculinity, they are its evolution. They show children that strength isn't rigid, and power isn't one-dimensional.

Building Emotional Resilience for the Journey Ahead

Becoming a father is like stepping onto shifting ground: joy, exhaustion, love, frustration, all rolled into one relentless cycle. Emotional resilience is your anchor. It's the ability to stay grounded in the chaos, to bend without breaking, and to keep showing up even when you feel like you're falling apart.

Resilience doesn't mean suppressing your emotions: it means facing them, naming them, and learning how to respond rather than react. It's pausing before yelling. It's laughing at the mess instead of drowning in it. It's the mental muscle that helps you recover from a bad day and show up fully the next.

One powerful way to build this resilience is to cultivate self-awareness. Know your triggers. Pay attention to the moments when your patience thins and your anxiety spikes. Name those feelings instead of numbing them. "I feel overwhelmed right now," is a sentence that can change your entire trajectory. Awareness turns emotional chaos into clarity.

Another tool is daily reflection. Take five minutes at the end of the day to ask yourself: What went well? What didn't? How did I handle stress? What would I like to do differently tomorrow? Over time, this small habit becomes a compass, guiding you through the emotional terrain of parenthood.

And most importantly, lean on your community. Whether it's a circle of dad friends, a parenting group, or a therapist, let others walk with you. Connection is a powerful antidote to burnout. You don't have to carry everything alone.

Resilience doesn't make you immune to exhaustion or doubt. It just means you trust yourself enough to navigate through it. It means recognizing your capacity to grow, to repair, and to start over. And that is exactly what your children need to see.

Building emotional resilience is not a one-time achievement, it's a daily practice, a mindset, and a set of habits that support your growth through the highs and lows of parenthood. It begins with cultivating practical and sustainable coping strategies. One of the most powerful ways to do this is by establishing healthy routines that bring a sense of predictability amidst the ever-changing landscape of fatherhood. These routines don't need to be grand or time-consuming. A simple morning ritual, like savoring a quiet cup of coffee while watching the sunrise, can ground you as effectively as a thirty-minute workout. Similarly, winding down the day with a bedtime routine can provide both you and your child with comfort and structure.

Another cornerstone of resilience is developing a mindset centered around gratitude and positivity. In the midst of sleepless nights or chaotic mornings, taking a few minutes to reflect on what went right can shift your entire outlook. A gratitude journal, where you jot down small victories or moments of joy, helps you stay anchored in what matters. These reflections act as gentle reminders that progress exists even in the messiest moments. It's not about ignoring the hard parts, it's about holding space for the good alongside the challenging.

Equally important is building and maintaining a support system. Emotional resilience grows stronger when nurtured by community. Connecting with others who are navigating the same terrain brings reassurance, perspective, and shared wisdom. Local meetups, parenting workshops, and online groups tailored to dads offer not only advice and tips but also camaraderie. In these spaces, vulnerability becomes a strength, and shared laughter over common struggles lightens the emotional load. These communities act as a mirror, reminding you that you're not alone and that your feelings are valid and understood.

Committing to personal growth is another key element of resilience. Becoming a father doesn't mean you stop growing as an individual. In fact, parenting can become a powerful catalyst for self-discovery and self-improvement. Setting personal goals, whether it's learning a new skill, reading a parenting book, or simply reflecting on your values, keeps your identity vibrant and engaged. Prioritizing self-care is essential here. Whether it's a daily jog, five minutes of quiet meditation, creative pursuits, or just carving out space for solitude, these practices replenish your energy and help you show up more fully for your family.

One tangible way to integrate all of these practices into daily life is by setting aside a few quiet minutes each evening for reflection. Ask yourself: *What went well today? What did I learn? What can I try differently tomorrow?* This habit turns each day into a learning opportunity, transforming challenges into stepping stones for growth. It helps you gain clarity, recalibrate when needed, and track your emotional journey with intention.

Sharing meaningful family rituals can also fortify emotional resilience. These rituals, whether they're long-standing traditions or newly created ones, offer consistency and comfort. A Friday night pizza dinner, weekend nature walks, or Sunday pancake mornings create moments of joy and togetherness. They help children feel safe and secure, and they give you, as a parent, a reliable touchstone in the rhythm of family life. These rituals aren't just "nice to have"—they are grounding practices that build connection and stability.

Emotional resilience is like a muscle: the more you flex it, the stronger and more adaptive it becomes. By creating healthy habits, nurturing your support system, and embracing personal growth, you're not just surviving fatherhood, you're thriving in it. And as you grow, so does the environment you create for your child. Your ability to stay present, respond with patience, and recover from setbacks models emotional intelligence in real time. Your child will learn what it means to meet life's challenges with grace not by your words alone, but through your daily actions.

This resilience also helps you stay grounded during the inevitable storms of parenting. It teaches your child that strength isn't about being unshakeable, it's about being able to bend without breaking, to feel deeply without losing your center. And in doing so, you create a home filled with emotional safety and authentic connection.

As you continue on this transformative path, remember: resilience is not about being perfect, it's about being present, being kind to yourself, and being open to learning every day. You're not just building a legacy of fatherhood rooted in love and strength; you're showing your children how to become emotionally resilient individuals themselves. And that is one of the greatest gifts you can give them.

Fathers are no longer confined to outdated roles: they are nurturers, guides, and co-architects of their family's emotional landscape. Every small moment of growth, every decision to show up despite the chaos, adds to the story you are writing, not only for yourself, but for the generation you are raising. Let that story be one of courage, compassion, and lasting connection.

Chapter 2: Connecting with Your Newborn

It was one of those rare, hushed afternoons when time itself seemed to pause. The kind of stillness that settles gently over the house, wrapping everything in a blanket of calm. I found myself in the nursery, sunlight spilling softly through the curtains, casting golden patterns across the floor. My newborn son lay sleeping in his crib, his breaths slow and rhythmic, his tiny chest rising and falling like the tide.

I sat beside him, mesmerized by the miracle of his presence. At some point, his small hand found mine, and without hesitation, his fingers curled around one of mine, clinging with a quiet urgency. That single touch stopped me in my tracks. In that simple, instinctive gesture, I saw his need, not for words, or toys, or anything grand, but for connection. Pure, immediate, human connection.

That was the moment I truly understood the power of touch. It wasn't abstract or poetic. It was real, and it was profound. Through touch, we speak the first language we ever learn: the language of love, safety, and belonging.

Skin-to-Skin: The Power of Connection

The first time my son was placed on my bare chest, skin against skin, I felt something shift inside me. His warm body settled into mine, and I could feel the beat of his heart sync with mine in an unspoken rhythm. In that moment, all the chaos of new parenthood, sleepless nights, endless questions, quiet fears, faded into the background. What remained was presence. Connection. A sense of anchoring that felt both ancient and immediate.

Skin-to-skin contact isn't just touching. It's a powerful physiological and emotional exchange. For a newborn, it offers critical regulation of body temperature, heart rate, and breathing. It soothes the startle reflex, calms crying, and recreates the safe, enveloping feeling of the womb. This touch, so simple, becomes the baby's first experience of the world as safe, warm, and responsive.

But it isn't just the baby who benefits. For a father, it's grounding. Skin-to-skin contact promotes the release of oxytocin, the "bonding hormone" that deepens emotional closeness and tempers stress. It gives anxious dads a kind of emotional scaffolding, a way to participate deeply in the early days, even when everything feels unfamiliar. When your baby lies against your chest, with only a diaper and a blanket to separate you from the world, something opens up. A door into the softest, most instinctive part of yourself.

Meaningful skin-to-skin contact involves more than just holding your baby. It's about intention and comfort for both of you. Whether sitting in a recliner or lying back in bed, find a position that supports your baby's head and neck while allowing their body to rest fully against yours. Strip them down to their diaper and drape a warm blanket over their back. It's often easiest during quiet windows, after feeding, early mornings, or during naptime. These are natural pauses in your day, and perfect opportunities for uninterrupted bonding.

Integrate skin-to-skin into daily routines during bottle-feeding, after nursing, or even after bath time. That warm transition from water to chest can soothe overstimulation and extend the sense of comfort. Over time, this daily rhythm becomes more than a habit, it becomes a ritual, a steady point of connection in the ever-changing terrain of parenthood.

This isn't just something for one parent to do. When both partners engage in skin-to-skin contact, it creates shared experiences that build unity in your parenting dynamic. Trade off sessions. Discuss them. Talk about how it felt, what you noticed in your baby, what emotions stirred in you. These small conversations become building blocks of understanding: about each other, and about how you're growing into your roles.

Include siblings and grandparents in the practice as well. With appropriate supervision and gentle instruction, even older children can engage in skin-to-skin time with their baby brother or sister. It becomes a way for them to express love, establish connection, and feel involved in this tender phase of life. For grandparents, it can be an incredibly healing experience, reigniting old memories while creating new ones.

Reflection: Capturing the Moments

Try keeping a small journal dedicated to these moments. Write down what you feel, before and after each skin-to-skin session. Note your baby's behavior, your own mood, the shifts you observe in your connection over time. These entries don't have to be perfect or poetic, just honest. Later, they become a powerful archive of growth, of bonding, of love expressed in the simplest and most human way.

Mastering Baby Cues: Understanding What Your Baby Needs

It's three in the morning, and the stillness of the night is broken by your baby's cries. You stumble out of bed, rubbing the sleep from your eyes, heart racing as you try to decode what's wrong. Is it hunger? Discomfort? Fatigue? In those early weeks, it can feel like you're trying to navigate a foreign country without a map. But here's the truth: your baby *is* communicating. You just need to learn the language.

Babies may not have words, but they are master communicators through movement, expression, and sound. One of the earliest signs you'll encounter is the **rooting reflex**, that gentle turning of the head and open mouth, as if they're searching. This is their way of saying, *"I'm hungry."* You might also notice them sucking on their fists or making soft smacking sounds, clear signs it's time to feed. Meanwhile, yawns, eye rubbing, and a distant gaze often signal that your baby is ready for sleep. The earlier you catch these cues, the smoother things will go for both of you.

The goal isn't just recognizing the signals but learning how to respond with care and intention. Fussiness doesn't always demand a bottle; sometimes, all it

24

takes is a warm embrace, a gentle rock, or a walk around the room with a soothing hum. Babies are incredibly responsive to your tone, your energy, your presence. When you align your responses with their cues, feeding them before hunger escalates to cries, or laying them down before exhaustion sets in, you build a rhythm that reduces stress and nurtures trust.

Each day offers subtle lessons. Maybe your baby tends to get drowsy right after a mid-morning feed, or their energy surges after a short nap. Paying attention to these patterns turns guesswork into something closer to instinct. One of the most powerful tools you can use is a **Cue Journal**. Write down what your baby does and how you respond. Over time, you'll see patterns emerge, clues that help you understand what your child needs *before* they have to cry out for it.

These notes become more than data; they reflect your growing confidence as a parent. You'll start to know when your baby is overstimulated or just needs a little downtime. You'll notice how certain times of day lend themselves to tummy time or a playful moment, while others are better for snuggles and rest.

As you get to know your baby's rhythms, you can structure your day to better match their needs. You might find that playtime is most effective after a light feeding or that your baby enjoys music in the afternoon but prefers silence before sleep. These little discoveries make daily life smoother and more joyful, not just for your baby, but for you, too.

Your growing fluency in your baby's cues doesn't just make parenting easier; it strengthens your bond. Your baby feels safe, seen, and understood, and you feel empowered, capable, and deeply connected.

Decoding baby cues is not a solo mission. It's a duet between you and your partner. Talk about what you've observed. Share insights like, *"I noticed she rubs her ears when she's sleepy,"* or *"He gets fussy when the room gets too bright."* This shared language fosters unity and helps avoid unnecessary stress or confusion.

Swapping roles now and then can also provide perspective. Maybe your partner handles bedtime while you do mornings, then switch. You'll both gain a better understanding of how your baby communicates with each of you individually, and how to adapt together.

Exercise: Cue Journal

Start small. Keep a notebook or use an app to jot down the day's cues. When did your baby seem hungry? What signals did they give? How did they act before a nap? How did your response work? This journal becomes a powerful tool for reflection and planning, and something you and your partner can review together. It also serves as a beautiful record of your growth as parents.

Take note of any unique cues your baby seems to reserve for you versus your partner. Maybe your baby gives you more direct eye contact or calms quicker in your arms. Reflecting on these distinctions deepens your understanding of your role in their world.

What once felt like confusing chaos will, with time and attention, become meaningful communication. You'll begin to hear the difference in your baby's cries, recognize the look in their eyes before they fuss, and respond with confidence and compassion. This is not just about meeting needs, it's about building a relationship rooted in mutual trust and understanding.

Every sound, every gaze, every tiny movement is a piece of a conversation. Your job is to listen with your heart and respond with presence. And in doing so, you'll create a connection that lasts far beyond infancy, a foundation for communication, empathy, and love.

Creating a Bedtime Bond: Nighttime Routines for Dads

As a dad, your role in the bedtime routine is more than just helpful, it's profoundly meaningful. These quiet nighttime hours offer some of the most intimate opportunities to bond with your baby. In the stillness of the evening, when the world slows down, the rituals you build together become a source of comfort, trust, and connection.

Bath time can be one of the most effective ways to wind down and connect. The warm water has a calming effect on your baby's body, easing them into a relaxed state. As you gently wash them and talk softly, they begin to associate your presence with safety and serenity. The playful splashes, the soft washcloth against their skin, your steady hands, all of it communicates love in a language they understand instinctively. This simple routine becomes a cocoon of closeness, anchoring your baby in security as the day draws to a close.

After the bath, a cozy cuddle in a soft towel or warm pajamas provides another layer of closeness. You might hold your baby against your chest, sway gently, or rock together in a quiet room. These quiet post-bath moments allow your baby to feel the rhythm of your heartbeat, hear your voice, and settle into the peaceful presence of your arms. It's during this time that your bond deepens, not through grand gestures, but through steady, loving consistency.

Reading bedtime stories is more than a tradition, it's an act of nurturing. Choose books with calming tones, rhythmic patterns, and gentle illustrations. These types of stories help your baby wind down without overstimulating them. Even if your baby doesn't yet understand the words, your voice becomes a comforting cue that sleep is near. Over time, these stories will build the foundation for language development, imagination, and a lifelong love for books. But more immediately, they're a soothing bridge between wakefulness and rest.

Not every night will unfold peacefully. Some evenings may be filled with crying, resistance to sleep, or frequent wake-ups. This is normal. During those times, your calm presence makes all the difference. Try gentle motions, soft rocking, rhythmic patting on the back, or a quiet lullaby in a dim room. These small acts mimic the sensations of the womb and offer familiar comfort.

When your baby wakes up hungry in the middle of the night, having a plan can make things smoother. Preparing bottles or feeding supplies ahead of time minimizes disruption. Likewise, diaper changes should be quick, gentle, and as quiet as possible, keeping lights low and stimulation minimal.

The right environment can significantly influence your baby's sleep quality. Consider soft ambient sounds like white noise or gentle lullabies to mask household noise and recreate womb-like familiarity. A comfortable room temperature, cozy pajamas, and a firm, supportive crib mattress are all small but essential details.

Adding a soft-glow nightlight or a slow-moving mobile can offer gentle stimulation without interrupting your baby's ability to wind down. Choose calming colors and patterns, nothing too bright or flashy, to maintain a tranquil space that feels safe and soothing.

Your participation in these nightly rituals does more than promote better sleep. It builds a powerful sense of security in your baby. Your presence becomes part of the rhythm of their world: steady, dependable, loving. Each night, as you rock, read, sing, or soothe, you're building emotional scaffolding that supports your child's sense of safety and connection. And it's not just about them, it's about you, too. These moments foster your own emotional connection to fatherhood, deepening your role in your child's life in ways that words can't capture.

Exercise: Nighttime Reflection

At the end of each week, take a few quiet minutes to reflect on your bedtime experiences with your baby. Ask yourself:

- How did I feel during these moments?

- Did my baby seem more relaxed or responsive to certain parts of the routine?

- Were there any signs of changes in sleep patterns or temperament?

- What adjustments might help improve our nighttime flow?

Write down your thoughts in a notebook or a notes app, whatever feels most natural. Also consider how flexibility plays into your routine. Babies grow fast, and their needs evolve. Staying adaptable while keeping certain elements consistent is the key to long-term success.

Observe, adjust, and grow with your baby. These nightly reflections not only help you tune in to their needs but also give you a deeper understanding of your own experience as a dad.

Your role in your baby's bedtime routine is far more than functional, it's foundational. Each gentle touch, whispered lullaby, and loving gaze becomes a thread in the fabric of their emotional world. These are the moments that shape your bond, build trust, and create a strong, secure start to life. Lean into them fully, and know that your presence is the very thing that helps them sleep peacefully at night, and feel safe in the world.

Making the Most of Paternity Leave: Deepening the Bond with Your Baby

Paternity leave is more than just a break from work, it's a rare and sacred window of time where the pace of life slows down just enough for you to fully immerse yourself in your new role as a father. This period offers a chance to connect with your baby in ways that shape your bond for years to come. Rather than letting the days blend into one another, consider approaching this time with intention and heart. Think of it as your baby's first chapter, and you get to help write it.

Start by creating a flexible plan that reflects your priorities. You don't need an hour-by-hour schedule, but having some loosely defined goals, like morning walks, solo baby time, or specific daily rituals can help structure your days meaningfully. Prioritize presence over productivity. Whether you're taking your little one on a peaceful stroll through the neighborhood, rocking them to sleep in the stillness of dawn, or simply gazing at their tiny features as they nap in your arms, these quiet moments hold incredible power. They anchor your connection in love and familiarity.

Taking an active role in daily caregiving is one of the most impactful things you can do during your leave. Tasks like diaper changes, burping, and bath time might seem basic on the surface, but they're truly moments of bonding in disguise. These small, consistent acts become a language of trust between you and your baby. They learn your voice, your scent, your rhythm. Every time you respond to a cry or softly soothe their fuss, you're saying, "I'm here. You matter."

Feeding time, whether you're bottle-feeding, helping prep for breastfeeding, or doing skin-to-skin contact afterward, is another sacred space for closeness. It's not just about nourishment; it's about connection, eye contact, and being fully present in the shared quiet. In those moments, you're not just tending to their needs, you're helping them feel safe and known.

Use your leave to create memories that go beyond routine. This might be as simple as introducing your baby to nature with short outdoor visits or documenting "firsts" in a photo journal or video diary. Those chubby cheeks covered in bubbles during bath time, the first time they grip your finger with surprising strength, or the quiet afternoons when they sleep on your chest, these are the seeds of tradition, the beginnings of your family's unique story.

A fun idea: start a "dad and baby" ritual, like a specific lullaby you always sing or a short morning walk. Over time, these actions become cherished traditions, bringing comfort and familiarity as your child grows.

Parental leave isn't just about bonding with your baby; it's also an opportunity to reflect on the changing shape of your family. Use this time to check in with your partner, talk about how you're each adjusting, what's working, what's not, and how you can support one another better. Conversations like these can help realign your parenting values and create a stronger, more united front as you step into this next chapter together.

Also, give yourself space to reflect on who you are becoming. Fatherhood transforms you, it deepens your empathy, redefines your priorities, and introduces a new rhythm to life. Journaling, meditating, or even having quiet solo moments can help you process the immense changes unfolding within you.

No one is meant to do this alone. Tap into support networks, whether they're local parenting groups, online communities, or even fellow dads in your friend circle. Sharing experiences, both joyful and frustrating, can be a huge relief. You'll find comfort in knowing that others are fumbling through the same feedings, diaper blowouts, and sleepless nights. Conversations with other parents often lead to invaluable insights, unexpected laughter, and a sense of belonging that makes this journey feel less overwhelming.

Chapter 3: Supporting Your Partner

Have you ever noticed how some evenings feel different, like the world has paused just long enough for you to hear your own thoughts? The kind where the hum of the refrigerator seems louder than anything outside. My wife and I found ourselves seated at the kitchen table, the remnants of dinner pushed aside, the baby finally asleep. In that gentle hush, she began to unpack her day: the laughter, the frustrations, the tiny triumphs, and the raw exhaustion of motherhood.

My first instinct was to step in, to fix things. To offer advice, propose solutions, make it better somehow. But as I watched her: her shoulders slightly slumped, her voice edged with weariness, it struck me that she wasn't asking for answers. She was asking to be heard. She needed a companion, not a consultant. What she needed most in that moment was a safe harbor, a witness to her experience.

Reflective Listening Strategies and Practices

Active listening is not a passive act. It is deliberate. Transformative. It means showing up with your full presence, not just your ears. It's more than nodding while waiting to speak. It's giving your undivided attention, locking eyes with sincerity, and turning away from screens and distractions. It's leaning in, literally and figuratively.

To listen actively is to signal that the other person's thoughts matter, that their words are not floating into an empty space but landing on someone who genuinely cares. It's using small affirmations, "I hear you," "That makes sense," "Tell me more" that encourage continued sharing. Active listening turns conversations into connection. It shifts the dynamic from problem-solving to soul-hearing, from "What can I do?" to "Who are you in this moment?"

Imagine each exchange as a thread, and each act of listening as a gentle weaving. Over time, this becomes a tapestry: not of solutions, but of shared understanding and emotional intimacy.

While active listening holds the space, reflective listening helps give shape to what's inside it. It's a deeper mirror. It allows your partner's words to echo back: not to be repeated, but to be rephrased with care, capturing the emotions beneath the surface.

When your partner says, "I can't do this anymore," responding with, "It sounds like you're feeling really overwhelmed and unsupported," validates not just the words, but the heart behind them. This simple act tells them: *I see you. I understand what this feels like for you.*

Reflective listening helps untangle complex emotions. It invites clarity and often opens the door to unspoken fears, hopes, and needs. It's not about interpreting, it's about illuminating.

Validation is the cornerstone of emotional connection. It tells your partner: *Your feelings are real. They're allowed. And I respect them.*

When someone says they're frustrated, dismissing it with a silver lining or redirecting it with advice can unintentionally isolate them. But saying, "That does sound really hard," or, "I can see why that would leave you drained," acknowledges their reality. It shows compassion without the pressure to fix. This kind of support fosters trust, deepens emotional intimacy, and affirms that both partners can show up authentically in the relationship.

We all want to ease the pain of those we love. But often, the instinct to fix comes from our own discomfort with witnessing struggle, not from our partner's need for a solution.

Letting go of the fix-it mentality is not an act of indifference, it's a profound expression of trust. Trust that your partner is capable, resilient, and not broken. Trust that what they need most is your presence, not your prescriptions. Sometimes, just sitting together in silence, holding space for what is, can be the most healing thing of all.

Over time, this practice builds emotional intelligence within the relationship. It transforms moments of tension into opportunities for connection. And it fosters a bond that thrives on depth, not surface-level solutions.

Healthy communication doesn't happen by accident, it is intentional. It requires nurturing. One of the most impactful habits you can build as partners is creating space for regular emotional check-ins. These don't have to be formal or lengthy. Sometimes, a simple question like, "How are you really doing today?" asked while folding laundry or sharing tea, is enough.

Establish specific times, perhaps during a quiet dinner or once the baby is down, to talk about how you're feeling, what you need, and what's shifting. Open dialogue reduces assumptions and prevents resentment. It also reinforces the idea that your relationship is a living entity, deserving of attention and care.

A powerful way to strengthen your listening skills is to start an **Active Listening Journal**. After a meaningful conversation, take a few moments to reflect: What did your partner share? How did you respond? What worked? What didn't?

Documenting these reflections helps sharpen your emotional awareness and provides insight into your communication patterns. Over time, you'll begin to see trends, moments where empathy unlocked connection, or where rushing to a solution short-circuited a deeper exchange. This mindfulness becomes a tool for growth, not just in your relationship, but in how you navigate all emotional landscapes in life.

Parenthood is a shared metamorphosis. As your baby grows, so do you, individually and as a couple. And in that evolution, communication becomes your compass. Presence, empathy, validation, these are the tools that help you navigate the unpredictable terrain of new parenthood.

It's not about getting everything right. It's about showing up. Fully. With open hearts and willing ears. It's about turning toward each other, again and again, even when you're tired, even when you don't have answers.

This journey isn't just about raising a child. It's about raising each other, into stronger, more connected versions of yourselves.

Shared Responsibilities: Building Balance in the Home

In the whirlwind of new parenthood, even the walls seem to whisper reminders of things undone, laundry piles, half-folded blankets, unopened mail. The weight of domestic responsibilities can easily tilt the scales, creating tension and burnout.

To avoid this imbalance, start with a clear conversation. Sit down and make a comprehensive list of daily and weekly tasks. Include everything, washing bottles, grocery planning, tidying up toys, late-night feedings, scheduling pediatric appointments. Then discuss how to divide these responsibilities based on your individual strengths and preferences. Maybe you enjoy cooking, while your partner prefers tackling the laundry. Aligning roles with natural inclinations promotes harmony and avoids resentment.

But remember, life with a newborn is anything but predictable. What worked last week might not this week. Revisit your plans often. Be flexible. Stay curious about each other's evolving needs. Maybe your partner needs a break from bath time duties or you'd like to take over bedtime for a few nights. These micro-adjustments, done with kindness, keep the relationship fluid and supportive.

Collaboration goes beyond task division, it's about shared ownership. Family check-ins, even brief ones, can help keep the emotional and logistical gears turning smoothly. Use these moments to brainstorm solutions together: "Would it help if we alternated night feedings?" "Should we try prepping meals for the week on Sundays?"

This kind of shared decision-making shifts the narrative from "Who's doing more?" to "How can we support each other better?" It builds solidarity. A partnership grounded in equity, not competition.

Sometimes, the best support comes from outside your immediate unit. And asking for help is not a sign of weakness, it's an act of wisdom. Whether it's hiring a cleaning service, ordering takeout more often, or accepting help from family and friends, these small acts of outsourcing can create massive relief.

There is no prize for doing everything alone. Your worth as a parent and partner isn't tied to how much you carry, it's tied to how present and connected you are. Leaning on your village, whether it's a friend who drops off a casserole or grandparents who babysit, frees up space for what truly matters: time with your baby, time with each other, and time to simply breathe.

Task Swap and Monthly Review: Building Empathy Through Shared Experience

Introducing a **Task Swap Exercise** can be a powerful tool in cultivating mutual understanding and balance. Begin by trading one daily task for a week, perhaps you take on morning bottle feedings while your partner handles the bedtime routine. At the end of the week, sit together for a moment of honest reflection. Discuss what you learned from stepping into each other's roles, what surprised you, what felt manageable, what felt overwhelming. These insights reveal the invisible labor behind everyday duties and deepen your empathy for one another.

To keep this process fluid and responsive, incorporate a **Monthly Review** session. Designate a quiet time, perhaps the first Sunday evening of each month to reassess how tasks are divided. Ask questions like: *Are these responsibilities still working for us? Has anything changed in our routines or energy levels?* These reviews should not be approached as performance evaluations but as a check-in to honor each other's evolving needs and contributions.

This intentional approach to responsibility-sharing helps ensure that no one partner becomes silently overwhelmed. It acknowledges that parenting is not a static state but a dynamic experience requiring flexibility and care. These practices make space for open dialogue, reduce resentment, and reinforce a sense of partnership.

True balance is not found in a perfectly even split but in a **mutual commitment to fairness, recognition, and adaptability**. When both partners feel seen and supported, the emotional weight of parenthood becomes lighter. It's not about perfection, it's about creating a rhythm where both partners can thrive, together.

Balancing household and parenting responsibilities is about more than just logistics, it's a daily expression of love, respect, and unity. When both partners engage with intention and care, it sends a powerful message: *We are in this together.* The goal is not efficiency, but connection.

A household built on **reciprocal support** fosters a culture of teamwork rather than silent obligation. Equal contribution doesn't mean doing the same things but investing equal energy and commitment. It also means recognizing when one partner may need more rest, more support, or simply more space. Flexibility ensures that responsibilities shift gracefully without resentment.

Parenthood is an ever-changing experience, and the strongest partnerships are those that evolve with it. Tasks may need to be renegotiated as sleep patterns shift, work schedules change, or new developmental stages emerge. The key is to stay in conversation, to check in, reassess, and reaffirm your commitment to supporting each other.

External support plays a vital role in this balance. Whether it's a weekly cleaning service, meal kits, or relying on a grandparent's help, seeking outside assistance is not a sign of weakness. It is a **strategic act of love**, protecting your energy so that you can be present for your partner and your child. Remember: lightening the load doesn't diminish your role, it enhances your capacity to show up where it truly matters.

Navigating Postpartum Emotions: Practicing Empathy Every Day

The postpartum period is a time of profound transformation, not just for the baby, but for the mother and the family as a whole. Physically, emotionally, and mentally, the terrain shifts rapidly. What once felt manageable may now feel monumental. What once brought joy may now evoke tears. These fluctuations are not a reflection of your partner's strength or spirit; they are the body's response to a radical metamorphosis.

Hormonal changes following childbirth often trigger **sudden mood shifts**, tearfulness, and feelings of being overwhelmed. Recognizing these as biological responses rather than personal failures is crucial. It prevents blame and nurtures compassion. Sometimes, simply naming the experience, "This is the postpartum wave" can diffuse tension and invite tenderness.

But empathy extends beyond observation. **Postpartum depression and anxiety** are real, and they often masquerade as irritability, numbness, or intense fatigue. Signs to watch for include persistent sadness, withdrawal from loved ones, loss of interest in things once enjoyed, or intense feelings of guilt. If these symptoms linger beyond two weeks, it's important to encourage your partner to seek professional support. This is not about fixing, it's about helping them access the tools they need to heal.

Your role during this time is not to solve but to hold space. Be a patient witness to their emotions. Resist the urge to advise or redirect. Sometimes, the most healing words you can offer are, "I'm here," or "You're not alone." These phrases, though small, create emotional anchor points in a stormy sea.

Support is also found in the quiet gestures: refilling their water bottle, rubbing their back during a cry, taking the baby without being asked. These moments speak volumes: they say, *I see you. I love you. I'm with you.*

Remember too, that caring for yourself is part of this equation. A depleted partner cannot be a supportive one. Carve out space for rest, connection with friends, or even a moment of stillness. Self-care is not selfish, it's part of the ecosystem of emotional health in your home.

Normalize emotional dialogue. Let your household be one where **feelings are not dismissed but welcomed**. Where tears aren't something to hide, and mental health is discussed with the same normalcy as physical health. When emotional safety is embedded in your home, it becomes a sanctuary, not just for now, but for the years to come.

These early months are not just about survival, they are about laying a foundation for the kind of relationship you want to model for your child. When they grow up in a home where empathy is practiced, where emotions are validated, and where care is mutual and dynamic, they learn not just how to give love, but how to receive it too.

Empathy is not a one-time act, it's a lifelong practice, an ever-expanding capacity. As you move through each new stage of parenting, revisit these principles. Check in with your partner. Ask, *How are you doing, really? What do you need right now?*

These questions, and the listening that follows, become the threads of a relationship woven with care and consciousness. A relationship that doesn't just weather change but is shaped and strengthened by it.

Let this be your intention: to parent not only with skill but with soul. To walk beside your partner with presence, curiosity, and compassion. To build a home where both of you, and your child, can feel seen, supported, and deeply loved.

Rebuilding Intimacy: Strengthening Your Relationship

The arrival of a newborn often brings immense joy, but also an unexpected disruption to the intimate rhythms of a relationship. What once felt spontaneous and seamless between partners can now feel strained or paused entirely. Physical exhaustion, emotional upheaval, and the sheer demands of caring for a baby can sap time, energy, and even the desire for closeness. But this shift doesn't signal loss, it signals evolution. Rebuilding intimacy in this phase isn't about returning to the way things were; it's about growing together in new, more resilient ways.

In the thick of midnight feedings and diaper duty, emotional intimacy becomes the bedrock. A gentle hand on the shoulder, a moment of laughter over spilled milk, or even just a shared glance across the room while soothing your child, these small gestures anchor the bond that still pulses quietly beneath the surface of parenthood's chaos. They're reminders that you are more than co-parents; you are partners navigating this wild, beautiful chapter together.

While candlelit dinners and spontaneous getaways may be temporarily off the table, intimacy doesn't have to vanish, it simply needs to be reimagined. Think cozy evenings with takeout and a favorite movie, or breakfast in bed while the baby naps. These moments don't have to be grand; they just have to be intentional. Even daily routines can hold powerful opportunities for reconnection. A shared morning coffee, folding laundry side by side, or brushing your teeth together at night can become quiet rituals of closeness.

Crucially, intimacy thrives on communication. This is a time to talk, not just about parenting strategies and nap schedules, but about how you're feeling, what you're missing, and what you need. Open, judgment-free dialogue allows both partners to express their desires, frustrations, and hopes. Vulnerability becomes a bridge, not a burden. By creating a space where emotional and physical needs are discussed without shame or defensiveness, couples can replace tension with understanding, and silence with supportive action.

Exploring new forms of intimacy beyond physical connection can also be a game-changer. Shared hobbies, like cooking, gardening, puzzles, or learning a new skill, can provide fresh ways to bond and rediscover each other. Even parenting milestones, such as surviving a sleepless week or celebrating baby's first giggle, can bring you closer. These shared victories remind you of the teamwork and unity at the heart of your relationship.

Remember: intimacy isn't just about sex: it's about presence, attention, and care. A warm embrace, a compliment, a sincere thank-you can reignite the spark. Scheduling time to talk without distractions, surprising your partner with their favorite snack, or simply offering a back rub after a long day, these acts speak volumes. They say: "I see you. I value you. I'm still here with you."

Rebuilding intimacy is not about recreating what once was, but constructing something more enduring, more attuned to your current realities and future aspirations. These efforts, however small, lay the groundwork for deeper connection. They don't just mend the cracks that stress and fatigue may create; they reinforce the foundation with care, patience, and renewed affection.

And when physical intimacy begins to return, let it be guided by comfort and mutual readiness, not pressure or timelines. Every couple's pace is unique. The most important thing is creating a safe, loving space where both partners feel desired and emotionally secure.

As you continue building your family, let this rebuilding phase be one of intentional tenderness and growth. Through flexibility, empathy, and daily connection, you'll discover that intimacy isn't lost, it's simply transformed.

In the next chapter, we'll explore how these strengthened bonds become the emotional blueprint for your parenting journey, helping you foster a home environment rooted in connection, compassion, and shared purpose.

Chapter 4: Handling the Home Front

It was a Saturday morning, but it didn't feel like the ones I remembered. The soft gurgle of our baby blended with the rhythmic hum of the coffee maker. Instead of leisurely flipping through the news or sipping a hot cup of coffee uninterrupted, I found myself in the kitchen, wearing an apron, cradling the baby monitor under one arm, and fighting back both the sting of onions and the slow wave of sleep deprivation. Cooking breakfast had somehow transformed into a mission-critical task that required strategic thinking, nimble hands, and near-silent execution to avoid waking the baby.

This was no longer about "getting things done." It was about adapting. In this new season of life, cooking and cleaning weren't just chores, they were lifelines to maintaining order, sanity, and connection. The home front had changed, and with it came a need to rethink how we managed the everyday.

Cooking and Cleaning: Your New Normal

For new dads, streamlining household routines isn't just a convenience, it's a way to create space for presence, for peace, and for partnership. Cooking, once an afterthought or a quick post-work scramble, now demands planning, precision, and purpose. But here's the silver lining: it can also be an expression of care.

Batch cooking becomes your best ally. Dedicate a few hours on a quiet Sunday to prepare multiple meals, think hearty chili, veggie-loaded pasta bakes, or slow-cooked shredded chicken that can be reused across dishes. Freeze these meals in portioned containers so that during the week, dinner becomes a simple matter of reheating, not reinventing. An Instant Pot or slow cooker turns into a quiet kitchen hero, giving you time back while still delivering warm, nourishing meals.

To break the monotony, explore **new recipes or global cuisines**. Turn cooking into a low-pressure adventure, try Thai curries one week, Greek salads the next. Let your kitchen be a classroom, a playground, and a meeting place. Even toddlers can join by handing you ingredients or sprinkling cheese, transforming what could be a solitary duty into a shared family experience. Imagine your little one squealing with joy while shaking a salad dressing jar or pressing dough with tiny hands. These small moments can become memories that anchor your days.

Let's be honest, keeping the house clean with a newborn is like trying to keep the ocean still. Just when you finish one task, three more emerge. And yet, a clean, semi-organized space offers mental clarity in a time when chaos is never far.

Instead of chasing perfection, **create a sustainable system**. Develop a rotating schedule, perhaps focus on bathrooms Monday, laundry Tuesday, and floors

Wednesday. Set a timer for 15-20 minute "power cleans," choosing one or two rooms and giving them a quick refresh. Even a small reset can restore a sense of control.

Invest in tools that save you time and energy: a cordless vacuum for those sudden spill emergencies, microfiber cloths for fast surface cleaning, and multipurpose, non-toxic cleaners that are safe around the baby. Think efficiency over perfection, your goal isn't a showroom-ready space, but a functional, comforting one.

You don't have to shoulder everything alone. In fact, inviting your partner and older children into the mix strengthens the family fabric. Assign simple, age-appropriate chores, toddlers can put toys in bins, preschoolers can help sort laundry, and older kids can set the table or sweep the kitchen. Present tasks as opportunities for teamwork and life learning.

Even more importantly, **reframe chores as connection**. Turn cleaning into a dance party, cooking into a group project, or folding laundry into a time for conversation. Shared domestic responsibilities not only ease the burden but create moments for bonding, laughter, and even gratitude. When your child proudly carries a folded towel to the bathroom, they feel needed, and you feel supported.

The temptation to keep everything pristine is understandable, but unrealistic. With a newborn, life is messy. There will be dishes in the sink, pacifiers under the couch, and baskets of unfolded clothes. And that's okay.

Instead of fixating on spotless counters, **focus on what matters most**: keeping the home livable, loving, and lighthearted. A bit of clutter is a sign of life happening. Choose peace over perfection. Spend that extra 15 minutes snuggling on the couch rather than scrubbing grout. Those are the moments that matter.

Interactive Element: The Family Meal Planning Chart

Try this fun, hands-on activity: **Create a family meal planning chart.** Use a whiteboard, poster board, or digital template where each family member contributes a meal idea or favorite dish. Add stickers, magnets, or drawings to make it fun for kids. Assign themes **"Meatless Mondays," "Taco Tuesdays," "Pasta Thursdays," or "Breakfast for Dinner Fridays"** to build anticipation and structure.

Rotate responsibility each week, maybe one child helps plan, while another helps prep. It builds inclusion, reduces decision fatigue, and turns mealtime into a collaborative event. Over time, these rituals become part of your family identity, a comforting rhythm amidst the unpredictability of parenting.

The beauty of this evolving "new normal" lies not in strict routines, but in the grace you give yourself, and the joy you discover in unexpected places. Cooking and cleaning no longer feel like chores when they become invitations to connect, create, and collaborate.

In those small daily acts, preparing a favorite meal, wiping tiny handprints off the walls, dancing with a broom in hand, you're not just maintaining a house. You're building a home. One filled with love, laughter, and the kind of quiet strength that carries your family forward.

Diaper Duty and Bath Time: Dad's Guide to Baby Care

There's a unique kind of magic in the daily rituals of baby care, hidden in the folds of a diaper and the gentle splash of bathwater. These seemingly mundane tasks become powerful moments of connection, teaching new dads not just how to care for a child, but how to *be present*.

Changing diapers may not be glamorous, but it's a badge of honor for any dad learning the ropes. It's a skill born from trial, error, and a sense of humor. The first step is to set up a well-stocked and functional changing station. Choose a stable surface, ideally with a padded changing mat, and make sure you have:

- Diapers (in bulk!)
- Unscented baby wipes
- Diaper rash cream
- A change of clothes
- A small toy for distraction
- A disposal bin or diaper pail within reach

This setup isn't just about convenience, it's about creating a calm, efficient space where you can focus on your baby, not fumble for supplies.

Technique matters too. Place your baby gently on the pad, secure them with one hand, and unfasten the diaper with the other. Always wipe front to back to avoid infections, and apply cream if needed. One pro tip: slide the new diaper under before removing the soiled one to minimize messes and reduce wiggle time. As you practice, you'll move with more confidence, maybe even a touch of flair.

But don't rush through it. These few minutes are perfect for cooing, singing a silly song, or simply sharing eye contact. Your calm demeanor becomes a source of comfort.

Bath time can be a highlight of your day, a warm, soothing ritual that wraps care and play into one experience. But it starts with preparation.

Before you even run the water, gather everything you'll need:

- A soft hooded towel
- A mild, tear-free baby shampoo and body wash
- A gentle sponge or washcloth
- A clean change of clothes and fresh diaper
- A plastic baby tub or infant bath support
- A cup for rinsing

Fill the tub with only 2-3 inches of warm water (test with your elbow, the water should feel comfortably warm, not hot). If possible, place the bath setup on a waist-high surface to avoid straining your back.

Use soft, deliberate motions to clean your baby, starting with their face and working your way down. Support their head and neck throughout, especially for newborns. Speak softly, sing a lullaby, or simply narrate your actions. Your voice becomes an anchor of security.

After the bath, swaddle them quickly in the towel and hold them close. There's something deeply soothing about that post-bath cuddle, warm skin against your chest, wrapped in softness and trust.

Parenting isn't always smooth. Diaper rash can appear suddenly, caused by moisture, friction, or sensitivity. To prevent and treat it:

- Change diapers frequently
- Let your baby's skin air out when possible
- Use a barrier cream with zinc oxide
- Avoid scented wipes or diapers that might irritate

If bath time becomes a battle, crying, flailing, or visible discomfort, take a step back. Start with sponge baths until your baby becomes more comfortable. Use toys, warm cloths, gentle music, or even take baths together to ease the transition. Turn it into play rather than a task.

These routines are goldmines for early learning. Diaper changes become chances to name body parts, describe textures, or count toes. Bath time becomes sensory play: exploring warm water, gentle bubbles, and floating toys.

Try these interactive touches:

- **Sing familiar nursery rhymes** during diaper changes
- **Narrate your actions**: "Now we're wiping your tummy, tickle, tickle!"
- **Introduce colors and counting** with bath

toys
- **Let them explore**: Soft cups, rubber ducks, or floating rings can become tools for motor development

These micro-moments of interaction enrich your baby's brain while deepening your bond.

Reflection Section: Start a Baby Care Journal

Create a space to document these intimate moments, your wins, your flubs, your child's little quirks. Jot down funny diaper mishaps, bath time discoveries, or new routines you're trying out. Over time, this journal becomes a treasure trove, a reminder of how far you've come and how much love has been poured into every swaddle and splash.

Scheduling Success: Managing Family Time and Chores

One morning, the sight of sunlight dancing across a floor cluttered with building blocks and baby clothes made me pause. Amid the chaos, a single thought emerged: *we need structure*. Not rigidity, but rhythm. Not a strict regimen, but flow.

Establishing a loose but dependable daily rhythm helps the whole household thrive. Start with anchor points:

- **Consistent wake-up and bedtimes**: Crucial for babies and older kids alike. Predictability helps them feel safe and rested.
- **Mealtimes together**: Whether it's breakfast

smoothies or sit-down dinners, eating together is a chance to reconnect.

- **Nap and quiet times**: Essential for little ones and a breather for you.
- **Playtime and outdoor breaks**: Fresh air changes everything.

Post a visual schedule on the fridge or a family board. For toddlers and preschoolers, include pictures so they can "read" the day too.

No need for Pinterest-perfect activities. What matters is consistency and connection:

- **Game night Mondays**: Pick a simple board game, even if you bend the rules.
- **Movie Fridays**: Pajamas, popcorn, and a favorite film.
- **Nature Saturdays**: Whether it's a trail, park, or backyard garden, movement in nature soothes minds and recharges spirits.

Even small rituals, like making pancakes on Sunday or reading books together every evening, become the glue that holds a family close.

Chores won't vanish, but they can become manageable. Use **time-blocking** to stay organized:

- **Morning block**: Tidy kitchen, do one load of laundry
- **Afternoon block**: Tidy play area, prep dinner
- **Evening block**: 15-minute speed clean before bed

Rotate responsibilities with your partner, and don't be afraid to ask for help.

Personal time matters, too. Block 30 minutes for a solo walk, reading time, or meditation. These mini-recharges allow you to show up fully, not just as a parent, but as *you.*

Together, diaper changes and family walks, bathtime giggles and chore charts, these aren't just parts of a routine. They're the heartbeat of your home. Through them, you're not only caring for your child but nurturing a whole new version of yourself as a father, one that's attentive, grounded, and beautifully human.

Incorporating quick stress-relief techniques into your family schedule can be a game-changer. Mindfulness exercises, such as deep breathing, gratitude journaling, or even short guided meditations, can create pockets of calm throughout the day. These small but powerful rituals help center your thoughts, reduce anxiety, and promote mental clarity. Even five minutes of stillness with your partner or child can bring a profound sense of peace. Consider introducing family meditation sessions or breathing exercises before bedtime to help everyone unwind and transition into rest. These shared moments of calm foster a nurturing household atmosphere, where emotions are acknowledged and gently guided toward balance.

Parenting isn't static, and neither should your schedule be. Life with children is in constant motion: growth spurts, sleep regressions, school events, and changing work demands all influence the daily rhythm. A successful schedule is one that evolves alongside your family. When major changes occur, like starting a new job, welcoming a new baby, or shifting school terms, re-evaluating your routine ensures it remains relevant and supportive. The key lies in maintaining open dialogue. Invite every family member, even the youngest, to voice their needs. This inclusivity not only encourages communication but also teaches respect and consideration from an early age.

Through trial and error, I've learned that an effective family routine isn't about perfection or rigid control. It's about creating a supportive framework, a guide that brings predictability to the day without suffocating spontaneity. Some days will follow the plan flawlessly, while others may fall completely off track. That's okay. What matters most is having a flexible mindset, one that prioritizes connection over control. When you're able to pivot with grace, you show your children that adaptability is just as valuable as discipline.

Tech-Savvy Balance: Using Digital Tools Wisely

Technology, when used intentionally, can be a helpful ally in maintaining structure. Digital calendars, reminder apps, and family organizer tools like Cozi or Google Calendar can streamline communication and coordination. Shared to-do lists, grocery plans, and event trackers eliminate confusion and keep everyone on the same page. However, like any tool, technology must be managed with care.

Set clear boundaries for screen time to preserve meaningful interactions. Designate areas in the home as tech-free zones, like the dining table, bedrooms, or reading nooks, where conversations and bonding take priority. Encourage your kids to engage in board games, crafts, puzzles, or nature walks instead of defaulting to digital entertainment. These moments of unplugged connection encourage creativity, imagination, and genuine family presence.

Using technology to support your schedule, not dominate it, keeps your household running smoothly while preserving the essence of what matters: togetherness.

The path to a balanced home life is paved with empathy, communication, and flexibility. When each family member feels heard and respected, the household becomes a cooperative, thriving space. Your schedule doesn't have to be flawless to be effective, it simply needs to reflect your values and serve your family's evolving needs.

As you grow into your role, you'll discover that success doesn't mean checking every task off a list. It's found in the laughter during dinner, the calm of a shared breath, and the comfort of knowing that your home is a place of love, safety, and support.

Designing a Dad-Friendly Home: Where Safety Meets Comfort

One afternoon, as I sat surveying our living room, I realized something crucial, our home needed a serious makeover. Not in a cosmetic way, but in a way that would make it a secure, comfortable space for a tiny new explorer. The toys, the coffee table corners, the accessible electrical sockets, they suddenly looked like obstacles on an obstacle course my baby would be eager to take on. And that's when it hit me: creating a dad-friendly home isn't just about childproofing; it's about reshaping your space with intention, love, and a little bit of elbow grease.

Let's start with the essentials. Babyproofing might sound overwhelming, but think of it as crafting a fortress where curiosity can roam free without worry. Begin with safety gates at the top and bottom of every staircase, those first wobbly crawls and steps need boundaries. Next, invest in outlet covers, because those little fingers find *everything*. Secure any top-heavy furniture: bookshelves, dressers, even your TV, to the wall. Babies are climbers-in-training, and you don't want your home turning into an unintended jungle gym.

Don't stop at the obvious. Check your houseplants: *are they non-toxic?* You'd be surprised how fast a leaf ends up in a mouth. Declutter floors and hallways for safer mobility, and make regular sweeps for choking hazards: small toys, loose change, forgotten buttons. These might seem like small things, but they make a world of difference in creating a space that says: "You're safe here."

Safety gets you peace of mind, but comfort is where you and your baby will really flourish. Start with the layout. Arrange furniture so you can easily see your baby from any room, especially those open play areas. It's not just about visibility, it's about *presence*, being part of their world even when you're folding laundry or sipping your first coffee in hours.

Design cozy corners with soft lighting, warm rugs, and inviting pillows. Think of these nooks as your family recharge zones, perfect for books, naps, or just lying on the floor and staring at the ceiling fan together. These pockets of comfort become your refuge on the long days, and even longer nights.

Don't forget to leave your personal touch. Your home should reflect *you*. Your values, your passions, your quirks. Set up a corner just for yourself: a reading chair, a mini workspace, a spot to decompress or catch up on work. Add photos of your childhood, trophies from your hobbies, or a few framed jerseys. This isn't just about aesthetics, it's a subtle invitation to your child: *This is who I am, and one day, you'll know these stories too.*

No matter how beautifully designed your home is, if it's not functional, it'll fall apart during crunch time. Think of organization as your behind-the-scenes superpower. Set up baby care stations around the house: a basket of diapers and wipes in the living room, a feeding caddy in the bedroom, spare pacifiers in the kitchen. You'll thank yourself during those 3 a.m. emergencies.

Having clear homes for toys, books, and baby gear keeps the house from feeling like a war zone. And it helps everyone: your partner, your baby's babysitter, even visitors, know where things go. Less clutter, less confusion, more calm.

The vibe of your home matters more than you think. Use color to set the tone, cool blues and greens for calm, playful yellows for energy. Incorporate soft textures in rugs, throws, and curtains that invite touch and comfort. Hang framed pages from your favorite children's books or prints that inspire storytelling and play.

And here's a pro tip: let your child add to the decor.

Whether it's finger-paint art or scribbled masterpieces, give them space on the walls. It tells them: *Your voice belongs here, too.*

Chapter 5: Maintaining Mental Wellness

Recognizing the Signs of Dad's Postpartum Depression

One evening, after an exhausting day, I found myself staring blankly into the refrigerator. I wasn't really looking for anything; I just stood there, lost in thought. The soft hum of the appliance became a kind of comfort as my mind buzzed with overwhelm. I felt detached, like I was watching my life from the outside. It wasn't until later that I realized these moments of disconnection and numbness were signs of something deeper.

Postpartum depression isn't exclusive to mothers; it can also affect fathers, often quietly, and in ways that are easy to overlook. It can make it difficult to bond with your baby or connect with your partner. Recognizing that men can experience postpartum depression is essential for supporting mental health during early parenthood.

Although most discussions about postpartum depression focus on mothers, research shows that fathers can suffer as well. A systematic review on paternal postpartum depression highlights symptoms in dads that often present differently than in mothers. Rather than sadness, men might experience irritability, anger, or even emotional numbness. They may feel overwhelmed by their new responsibilities, wrestle with feelings of inadequacy, and carry unspoken guilt. These emotions can strain your relationships and create a sense of distance from the very family you've worked so hard to support.

Early recognition is key. Watch for signs that go beyond typical new-parent stress. Persistent sadness or irritability that doesn't ease up, a tendency to withdraw from loved ones or activities you used to enjoy, changes in appetite, or disrupted sleep, these are all potential indicators. If these symptoms persist and begin to interfere with everyday life, they may signal postpartum depression.

It's important to understand that depression is not a personal failing. It's a medical condition, one that is treatable. Research suggests that about 1 in 10 new fathers experience postpartum depression (Paulson & Bazemore, 2010). That statistic alone emphasizes the need for awareness and open conversation.

Distinguishing between normal stress and depression can be difficult. Stress may leave you feeling exhausted, but still able to function. Depression, however, can drain your energy and motivation, making everyday tasks feel overwhelming. The duration and intensity of your feelings matter. If symptoms last more than a few weeks or begin to worsen, it's time to consider seeking help.

Early intervention is essential for your own well-being and for your family's stability. Start by having an honest conversation with your healthcare provider. They can help determine whether what you're experiencing is stress or depression and guide you toward the right treatment. Options may include therapy, medication, or a combination of both. Therapy, in particular, offers a safe, non-judgmental space to explore your thoughts and develop healthier ways to cope.

Many therapists who specialize in paternal postpartum depression use cognitive behavioral therapy (CBT), which focuses on identifying and changing negative thought patterns. Group therapy can also be incredibly helpful, connecting with other fathers going through similar struggles can ease feelings of isolation and foster emotional resilience.

Self-Reflection Checklist: Are You Struggling with Postpartum Depression?

Take a few minutes to assess your mental health with the following questions:

- Are you experiencing persistent sadness, irritability, or mood swings?
- Have you lost interest in activities you used to enjoy?
- Have your sleep or eating patterns changed significantly?
- Do you often feel tired or drained, even after rest?
- Are you withdrawing from your partner, child, or social life?

Physical symptoms like fatigue or body aches can also be related to mental health. If these signs feel familiar, it might be time to consider that you're dealing with more than just new-parent stress.

Remember: reaching out for help is not a sign of weakness, it's a step toward healing. The sooner you address these symptoms, the sooner you can begin to feel like yourself again. This also strengthens your ability to be fully present for your child and partner, fostering a healthier home environment.

Coping with Stress and Anxiety: Simple Techniques That Help

One night, after a day packed with feedings, diaper changes, and no time for myself, I had a moment of clarity: I needed a way to manage the stress. Not just for me, but for my family. Taking small moments each day to reset made all the difference.

Try starting your morning with just a few minutes of deep breathing: inhale slowly through your nose, hold it briefly, then exhale through your mouth. That single act can calm your nervous system and give your mind a moment of peace. Meditation is also a powerful tool. Even 10 minutes of focused mindfulness can create space in your day to decompress.

You can also explore different meditation styles that suit your needs. **Guided visualization** helps you mentally escape to a calming scene, reducing stress through imagination. **Body scan meditation** shifts your focus inward, helping you become more aware of physical sensations and release tension gradually.

These practices are simple but powerful ways to build resilience. Over time, they can improve your mental clarity and emotional balance, something every parent deserves.

Physical activity is a powerful stress reliever. Whether it's a brisk walk around the block or a short yoga session, moving your body can help clear your mind and release built-up tension. You don't need to train for a marathon, simple, consistent movement can boost your mood and energy. Think of exercise as a deposit into your mental wellness account. The return? Increased clarity, emotional resilience, and improved well-being.

Cognitive behavioral techniques are another effective tool for managing stress and anxiety. Start by recognizing unhelpful thought patterns, the inner critic that whispers doubt or fear. Challenge those thoughts with facts and logic. If you find yourself thinking, "I'm not cut out for this," try reframing it: "I'm still learning, and that's okay." Practicing mindfulness can also anchor you in the present, preventing your thoughts from spiraling into worry. It's about focusing on what's happening now, rather than what might go wrong.

Positive affirmations can help shift your mindset over time. Repeating simple, encouraging statements like "I am capable" or "I grow with each experience" can reinforce your strengths and cultivate self-compassion. These reminders gently rewire your thinking, helping you approach fatherhood with more confidence and calm.

Effective time management is essential for reducing stress. Begin with a prioritized to-do list and break larger tasks into smaller, manageable steps. There's satisfaction in checking things off, and each small win adds up. Don't hesitate to delegate tasks: ask your partner, involve your family, or seek outside help. Lightening your load gives you more space to focus on what truly matters.

Professional support can be invaluable. Speaking with a therapist, especially one who specializes in parental mental health, offers tailored strategies for navigating stress and emotional challenges. Therapy isn't only for crises, it's a proactive way to build self-awareness and resilience. You might also benefit from parenting workshops or stress management programs, which can provide practical tools and fresh perspectives.

Finding Your Support System: Dads' Groups and Beyond

Discovering your support network is like finding a lifeline. When I first joined a group of fellow dads, I felt out of place, unsure of what to expect. But as we talked, I realized we were all facing similar challenges. The value of connecting with other fathers became immediately clear. It was comforting to know I wasn't alone in the sleepless nights and chaotic diaper changes. That sense of camaraderie, of being truly seen and understood, was emotionally grounding.

Beyond emotional support, these groups offer valuable insight and learning opportunities. Hearing how others handle parenting situations can introduce new strategies and ways of thinking you may not have considered.

Finding these groups might feel intimidating at first, but they're more accessible than they seem. Start by looking up local dad meetups or parenting clubs in your area. Many communities host regular gatherings at libraries, community centers, or even in someone's home. If in-person meetings aren't your thing, try joining an online dads' forum. These platforms let you connect, share advice, and find support on your own schedule, no pressure, just connection.

Don't overlook informal relationships either. Friends or family members who are also new parents can be incredible sources of support. Organize playdates or casual get-togethers where you can talk, share experiences, and support each other. These connections often grow into lasting friendships that continue beyond the early parenting years.

You can also tap into **community resources**. Parenting workshops, support hotlines, and family services can help you gain knowledge and practical skills while connecting you with others in similar situations. Topics might include everything from infant care to communication with your partner, and these programs are often welcoming and inclusive.

Lastly, the **diversity within parenting communities** can be an unexpected gift. Engaging with fathers from different cultural or social backgrounds broadens your perspective. You'll gain insights into alternative parenting styles and traditions that may inspire and enrich your own approach to fatherhood.

Prioritizing 'Me Time'

Taking care of yourself is not selfish, it's essential. Prioritizing "me time" safeguards your emotional and mental well-being, allowing you to show up more fully for your family. Consider self-care non-negotiable. Set clear boundaries to protect your personal time, and don't feel guilty for taking it. Think about what recharges you: reading, a favorite hobby, a quiet moment with coffee, and make it part of your regular routine.

Balancing personal time with family needs requires open communication and a bit of flexibility. Talk with your partner about carving out space for individual downtime. A well-planned schedule that includes both self-care and family time ensures no area of life gets neglected.

To make self-care sustainable, set realistic goals. Track your progress and be willing to adapt as life changes. What works now may shift as your child grows, and that's okay. The goal is to keep your own well-being on the radar, always.

Incorporating these habits into daily life builds emotional strength and stability. Over time, you'll find yourself better equipped to handle stress, navigate challenges, and support your family with clarity and compassion.

Interactive Element: Support Network Map
Create Your Support System

Start by building a *Support Network Map*. List all the people and resources available to you: local parent groups, online communities, friends, family members, and nearby support services. This visual helps you see your current support system and pinpoint areas where you may want to strengthen connections.

Why Support Matters

Fatherhood is a major transition, and having a strong support network can make all the difference. Connecting with others who understand your journey brings emotional relief and shared wisdom. Whether you find a local dads' group, attend meetups, or join online forums, these spaces offer camaraderie, advice, and a sense of belonging.

Every Connection Counts

Support doesn't always have to be formal. Talking with friends, reaching out to family, or participating in community workshops can be just as valuable. These interactions reduce the isolation many new fathers feel, improve mental health, and strengthen family relationships.

A Shared Journey

Fatherhood is not meant to be a solo path. Embrace opportunities to connect. The relationships you build contribute not only to your well-being but also to the emotional resilience of your entire family.

The Importance of 'Me Time': Recharging Through Self-Care

Why It Matters

In the chaos of early parenthood, taking care of yourself might feel like a luxury, but it's not. It's essential. Prioritizing your mental and emotional health helps you become a more present and effective partner and parent. Think of it like putting on your own oxygen mask first, you need to be well in order to support others.

What Recharges You?

Identify the activities that help you relax and feel energized. Maybe it's reading, listening to podcasts, woodworking, or jogging. Whatever brings you peace, make time for it. These activities aren't just distractions, they help you process emotions, think clearly, and reset mentally.

Make It a Routine

Balance between personal needs and family life takes planning and open communication. Talk with your partner about carving out personal time, maybe by swapping child care shifts or rearranging schedules. Treat self-care as a necessary part of your week, not something that only happens when there's time left over.

Fuel Your Body, Too

Eating well plays a big role in self-care. Nutritious meals and snacks can boost your energy and mood. Keep healthy, quick options on hand to stay fueled during busy days.

Sustainable Self-Care

Don't view self-care as a once-in-a-while indulgence. Make it part of your everyday life. Set achievable goals, like ten minutes of daily meditation or a weekly workout, and adjust as needed. Your routine should evolve with your changing schedule.

Interactive Element: Self-Care Plan Template
Use a simple template to create your *Self-Care Plan.*
- List daily, weekly, and monthly activities that bring you joy and relaxation.
- Add notes about what helps you recharge.

- Include new activities you want to try, exploring new interests can be revitalizing.

Tip: Spend time outdoors whenever you can. A short walk in nature can reduce stress, lift your mood, and leave you feeling grounded.

Taking time for yourself isn't selfish, it's vital for your well-being and your family's health. When you care for yourself, you create a more stable and loving home environment. These habits set the tone not just for your own life, but for your children's future too. By modeling healthy balance and self-care, you show your kids how to lead grounded, fulfilling lives.

Chapter 6:
Navigating Work-Life Balance

Setting Boundaries at Work: Protecting Family Time

There I was, once again working late, staring at the clock as the minutes ticked by. My phone buzzed. Just a picture, but one that hit me hard. It was my little one, grinning with that toothless smile that could light up a room. In that instant, I realized I was missing out on moments I'd never get back. Something had to change. Balancing work and family wasn't just a goal, it was a necessity. Creating boundaries at work became the key to preserving my family time without compromising my career.

Understanding the Power of Boundaries

Boundaries act as invisible guardrails, keeping work from seeping into personal life. Without them, the line between your professional and family roles can blur, leaving you overextended and disconnected. You may first notice it when you're mentally absent at dinner or constantly checking your phone. Recognizing these signs of imbalance is the first step. The next is clearly communicating your needs, letting your team and supervisors know that while your job matters, so does your family.

Practical Steps to Set and Maintain Boundaries

Start by defining your work hours, and commit to them. Avoid letting work spill into your evenings and weekends unless truly necessary. Use tools like email filters, auto-responders, and phone settings to limit interruptions outside of work hours. This helps you create a clear divide between work and home life. Schedule dedicated family days or downtime, and mark them on a shared calendar. Making these times visible and non-negotiable reinforces their value, for you and your family.

Involving your family in this process can also strengthen your efforts. Sit down together to create a balanced schedule that reflects everyone's needs. When your family feels included, they're more likely to support and respect the boundaries you've set.

Communicating with Colleagues Respectfully

Boundary-setting doesn't require confrontation, it requires clarity. Let your coworkers know your availability and when you'll be off the clock. This helps manage expectations and reduces pressure to respond immediately. A simple out-of-office reply or shared calendar can effectively signal your commitments without having to justify them.

Of course, boundaries will occasionally be tested. If someone crosses a line, respond calmly but firmly. You might say, "I understand this is important, but I'm unavailable after 6 PM due to family time. Can we reconnect first thing tomorrow?" Reaffirming your boundaries helps normalize them within your workplace. And if challenges continue, don't hesitate to seek guidance from HR or management, they're there to support a healthy work environment.

The Role of Leadership and Culture

Workplace culture plays a big role in boundary-setting. Pay attention to how leadership manages their own balance. If managers respect their personal time and encourage others to do the same, it sets a powerful example. Participating in mentorship or peer-support groups can also provide inspiration and practical tips for managing work-life balance effectively.

Reflection Exercise: Practicing Boundaries

Take a moment to write down your current work boundaries. Are they being respected? Reflect on times when those boundaries were tested, how did you respond? What might you do differently next time? This exercise helps you identify gaps and fine-tune your approach. Visualizing how you'd handle future challenges can also build your confidence in reinforcing those limits when needed.

Consider scheduling regular check-ins with yourself, maybe once a month, to reassess your boundaries. As your job responsibilities or family needs shift, your boundaries may need to evolve too. Staying flexible ensures that your system continues to serve you well.

The Ongoing Work of Balance

Balancing work and family isn't a one-time fix, it's an ongoing practice. As your children grow and your career progresses, your approach may need to shift. By setting clear boundaries, communicating them with respect, and adjusting as needed, you create a life where both career and family can flourish. You don't have to choose one over the other, you just have to be intentional about how you protect and prioritize both.

Remote Work and Parenting: Finding Harmony

The morning sun streamed through the window, lighting up the corner of my living room that now served as my office. Remote work had become the norm, offering flexibility but demanding discipline. My first step was to create a dedicated workspace, separate from high-traffic family areas. Whether it was a corner of the guest room or a quiet basement nook, having a defined area helped signal to everyone, including myself, that I was in work mode.

Investing in ergonomic furniture made a big difference. A comfortable chair and proper desk setup reduced physical strain and boosted focus. Productivity thrives in a space that's both functional and comfortable. Good lighting and sound control also played a key role in staying focused and minimizing distractions.

Balancing work tasks with parenting was the next big hurdle. Time-blocking became essential. I assigned specific hours for work and family, which brought structure and peace of mind. Knowing when to be fully present for each role helped me avoid the guilt of neglecting either. My partner and I coordinated shifts, while one worked, the other handled parenting, swapping as needed. Regular check-ins helped us adjust our schedules and support each other better.

To manage interruptions, we created simple cues, like a "do not disturb" sign or even a work hat, so family members knew when I needed focus time. Scheduled breaks allowed me to reconnect with my children intentionally. These pauses weren't just for rest, they were moments to engage, reminding them (and myself) that family came first. We also found activities, puzzles, crafts, or educational games, that kept the kids entertained during work hours.

Technology became a helpful tool in maintaining this balance. Task management apps and break reminders kept things on track. A shared digital calendar let the whole family know when I was working, helping everyone plan accordingly.

Flexible work arrangements offered both relief and challenge. By negotiating alternative hours or compressed workweeks, I was able to shape my schedule around our family's routine. This required open dialogue with my employer and a foundation of trust. Sometimes that meant working early mornings or late evenings so afternoons could be spent with the kids. The key was creating a consistent routine that worked for our family, even if it looked different from the traditional 9-to-5.

Remote work and parenting is an ongoing process of adapting and refining. It's not about getting it perfect, it's about making steady progress. With thoughtful planning, honest communication, and a willingness to adjust, you can build a sustainable routine that supports both your career and your family. Stay flexible. What works today may need to evolve tomorrow.

Making the Most of Commuting: Transitioning Between Roles

The daily commute is often treated as a time-consuming necessity, something to endure rather than enjoy. Yet with a shift in perspective, this stretch of time can be transformed into a meaningful opportunity for personal growth and connection. Whether you're on a packed train, stuck in traffic, or strolling to work, your commute can serve as a powerful tool for self-improvement, relaxation, and family bonding.

Instead of letting the time pass in idle frustration, consider engaging your mind through **audiobooks or podcasts**. These audio experiences can introduce you to new concepts, sharpen your skills, or immerse you in a compelling story. From professional development in fields like business, finance, or parenting to the calming escape of fiction, this simple habit turns idle time into an intellectual retreat. You arrive at your destination more informed, more inspired, and sometimes even more relaxed.

If your preference leans toward peace and quiet, your commute can also become a sanctuary for **mindfulness or meditation**. Practicing simple breathing exercises, tuning into a guided meditation, or just observing your surroundings without judgment can center your thoughts and reduce anxiety. By associating this practice with specific triggers, like a certain song, landscape, or even a particular bus stop, you train your mind to shift into a calmer state more quickly and consistently. This creates a buffer between the demands of work and the comforts of home, allowing you to arrive with emotional balance.

As the commute nears its end, it's essential to start mentally **transitioning from work mode to home life**. Use this time to review your day, not in a stressful way, but reflectively. Consider what you accomplished, what can wait until tomorrow, and what you're grateful for. Let go of lingering worries so you can cross the threshold into your home with a clear mind and an open heart. **Set a positive intention** for the evening: imagine greeting your children with enthusiasm, enjoying an unhurried dinner, or curling up for a bedtime story. These small, mental rehearsals prime you for presence, turning routine reunions into cherished moments.

You might also experiment with **different commuting methods** to enhance both your efficiency and well-being. **Carpooling with coworkers** can lead to meaningful conversations and shared experiences while also reducing your carbon footprint. **Public transportation** offers the luxury of passive travel, giving you the chance to plan, read, or just unwind. If geography allows, **walking or biking** injects physical activity into your day, promoting health, boosting mood, and sometimes unlocking creative insights that wouldn't surface in a car.

Technology can also be an ally in deepening **connections with family during your commute**. A quick check-in call, a funny photo, or a short voice note shows your loved ones they're on your mind, even when you're apart. These small gestures nurture closeness and signal that family remains a top priority despite the bustle. Sharing updates, like weather hiccups or traffic delays, invites them into your world and provides conversation starters later. These moments keep the emotional thread strong, weaving presence into absence.

In the end, **your commute doesn't have to be dead time**. With just a few mindful adjustments, it can become one of the most enriching parts of your day, a time to grow intellectually, prepare emotionally, and connect deeply. By reshaping this daily habit with intention and creativity, you transform it into a vital ritual that enhances both your personal life and your relationships.

Career and Fatherhood: Planning for Long-Term Success

Fatherhood has a way of rearranging your inner compass. Priorities that once dominated your focus, career advancement, status, long hours, may now take a back seat to something more profound: being present for your child's milestones, bedtime routines, and everyday joys. This new perspective doesn't mean giving up ambition, it means redefining success in a way that aligns with your evolving values.

Start by **re-evaluating your career goals**. Ask yourself: *Does my current path support the kind of life I want for my family?* If the answer is no, it might be time to explore career trajectories that allow for greater flexibility, meaningful engagement at home, and long-term fulfillment. This could mean seeking roles with more autonomy, shifting industries, or even starting your own business to gain control over your time.

Developing a **career-family integration plan** is a powerful step toward balancing professional drive with parental presence. Rather than treating career and family as competing forces, this plan helps you align them. Set milestones that respect both your professional development and your family time. Choose certifications or learning paths that offer remote access or shorter commitments. Prioritize work environments that understand and support the dual identity of worker and parent.

Remember, this plan should evolve with you. As your child grows, your career goals may change too. Review and revise this plan regularly, making sure it reflects both your aspirations and your family's needs. This living document becomes a guidepost, not a rigid blueprint, for sustainable success.

Think about **the legacy you're building through your career choices**. Beyond paychecks and promotions, what messages are you sending your children about values, integrity, balance, and purpose? Your choices become part of the life lessons they absorb. Modeling intentional, values-driven career decisions can leave a lasting impression that shapes how they one day navigate their own aspirations.

Don't overlook the resources your workplace may offer. **Family-friendly policies** like parental leave, flexible schedules, and remote work options can make a significant difference. If these benefits are available, use them. Fully embracing paternity leave, for example, not only strengthens your bond with your child but sets the tone for shared parenting. If your workplace lacks these policies, consider becoming an advocate. Speak up for initiatives that better reflect today's work-life realities, not just for yourself, but for others in similar shoes.

Connect with other working fathers. You're not in this alone, and community matters. Find or create peer groups that allow you to share strategies, vent frustrations, and celebrate wins. Attend seminars, parenting circles, or networking events designed for parents juggling multiple roles. These shared experiences foster camaraderie and offer practical advice rooted in real-life scenarios.

As you conclude this chapter on balancing career and fatherhood, hold onto this truth: **success is more than a title or salary**. It's the ability to be present for the moments that matter, to build a career you're proud of, and to raise children who feel seen, supported, and inspired. Align your goals with your values. Revisit your plans regularly. Use available resources and build a network of support. These are not just survival strategies, they're pathways to a richer, more rewarding life.

Keep communication open at home. Encourage regular family meetings to share plans, discuss goals, and celebrate progress. When your children see you prioritizing both your work and your time with them, they learn that balance is not only possible, it's worth striving for.

With clarity, intention, and heart, you can navigate the dual paths of career and fatherhood not as separate identities, but as **two powerful roles that enhance and strengthen one another**.

Chapter 7: Understanding Baby Development

The First Smile: Celebrating Early Milestones

It happened one golden afternoon, sunlight pouring gently through the window like a blessing. I was cradling my newborn daughter, her tiny frame curled against my chest, when she looked up at me. Her eyes: clear, searching, impossibly wise, locked with mine. And then, as if guided by magic, her lips curled into the faintest, most miraculous smile.

In that instant, time slowed. The world outside faded. It felt as though the universe itself held its breath to witness that sacred moment. That smile wasn't just a reflex, it was her first conversation with the world. A whisper of recognition. A glimmer of her inner light emerging. It changed everything.

For a new parent, moments like these are not just milestones; they're soul-markers. That tiny smile told me she was beginning to see me, not just as warmth and comfort, but as someone *known*. It signaled the awakening of her social spirit, the very beginning of her emotional landscape unfolding.

These early milestones, smiles, coos, the flutter of recognition in a baby's gaze, are more than developmental boxes to tick. They are threads in the fragile yet powerful tapestry of bonding. A baby's first smile says, *I see you. I trust you. I'm ready to connect.* It strengthens the invisible bond between parent and child and plants the seed of emotional security from which all future relationships will grow.

To honor these fleeting moments, consider capturing them in a milestone journal. Each entry, scribbled feelings, a photo, a date, becomes a sacred record, a love letter to your baby's journey. One day, when your child is older, you'll leaf through these pages together and feel those first sparks all over again. Invite family to be part of these celebrations, even through a video call or a quiet family dinner. These shared joys ripple outward, cradling your baby in a nest of love and belonging.

Your baby communicates from the very beginning, not with words, but with soft coos, fluttering eyelids, and those life-altering smiles. Every time you respond, by smiling back, by whispering softly, by holding their gaze, you're saying, *You matter. I'm here.* These are not small acts. They are the foundation of trust, the first bricks in the house of love you are building together.

Of course, not every day glows with magic. Some days feel like a blur of cries, fatigue, and self-doubt. When milestones seem delayed, or exhaustion weighs heavy, patience becomes a lifeline. Remember: every baby writes their own timeline. A missed milestone is not a failure. Even a single coo or a curious glance is a victory worth celebrating. Connecting with other parents, whether in a support group or over coffee, can ease the pressure and remind you: you're not alone in this.

It's easy to compare. To wonder why someone else's baby rolled over first or smiled more often. But development isn't a race, it's a bloom, and each child unfolds in their own time. If ever in doubt, a gentle check-in with your pediatrician can offer reassurance.

These visits aren't just checkups; they're opportunities to gain peace of mind, tailored guidance, and the clarity to focus on what matters most, your unique, precious child.

Milestone Reflection Prompt:

Try carving out a few quiet moments each week to reflect. What new things did your baby do? How did it make you feel? What did you learn about your baby, and about yourself? This ritual invites mindfulness, helping you stay grounded in the here and now, even as you marvel at the days flying by.

You might also dream ahead, imagine the next giggle, the first steps, the joyful chaos of their first word. This kind of reflection isn't just sweet, it helps you notice subtle changes and respond with the love and attention that nurtures growth.

Milestones like the first smile remind us that parenting is, at its heart, a collection of miracles tucked into the ordinary. These tiny triumphs build the emotional scaffolding of your child's world, and yours. They aren't just signs of development. They're reminders that love is growing, trust is deepening, and life, this beautiful, unpredictable life, is unfolding before your eyes.

Tummy Time and Beyond: Building Little Muscles and Big Confidence

Think about this: your baby, belly down, fists clenched in determination, eyes focused on the toy just out of reach. With every effort to lift their head, their tiny body wobbles like a sapling in the wind, but they don't give up. This is tummy time: a miniature workout and a bold declaration that they're ready to rise.

It may seem simple, but these moments are powerful. Tummy time helps strengthen the neck and shoulder muscles your baby will rely on to roll, sit, crawl, and eventually take those first unforgettable steps. It also helps shape their head, reducing flat spots and encouraging movement variety. Each time they push upward, they're not just building strength, they're building confidence.

But tummy time doesn't have to be a battle. Make it a playful invitation instead. Lay out colorful toys. Place a mirror nearby so they can marvel at their own reflection. Even your face, smiling, encouraging, can be their favorite motivation. Keep sessions short and sweet, cradling them into daily rhythms like post-nap cuddles or diaper changes.

At first, they may fuss. That's okay. With consistency and love, the floor becomes a space of discovery, a playground of possibility. And in these simple yet profound moments, you'll witness the beginning of their courage, one lift, one giggle, one wobble at a time. There's something truly heartwarming about the sight of your baby lifting their head during tummy time, tiny arms trembling with effort, eyes wide with wonder, their entire being focused on one brave push into the world. Now, imagine adding a gentle melody to that moment, a soft, soothing tune that wraps around the both of you like a lullaby in motion. Music has the power to elevate these simple exercises into magical experiences. A slow, rhythmic song can calm their spirit while encouraging gentle movement, turning tummy time into a dance of discovery and delight. Infant-friendly songs are more than just background noise; they become cues for play, invitations to wiggle, and comfort in times of effort. The right soundtrack can light up your baby's senses, making the floor their very first stage for movement and exploration.

As the days pass, each physical milestone becomes a testament to their quiet strength and growing independence. The first time they roll over, unassisted and unexpected, your heart may skip a beat. These small triumphs, recorded in a notebook or captured in a spontaneous photo, transform into priceless chapters in the story of their growth. Watching them scoot with determination toward a favorite toy is like witnessing the earliest sparks of their will and personality.

Encouraging this movement can be as simple as a well-placed toy, just out of reach, close enough to excite, far enough to challenge. And when they finally get there, the look of pride on their face mirrors the awe in your own.

But the play doesn't stop there. Beyond tummy time, there's a world of gentle activities that nurture both body and bond. Baby yoga and light stretches offer a beautiful opportunity to move together, skin to skin, heart to heart. These moments on a soft mat are more than physical exercise, they are shared rituals of closeness, grounding your connection in laughter, eye contact, and touch.

Playtime can continue into the bath, where water becomes a joyful playground. The splashes, the floating toys, the feel of water cascading down tiny arms, these sensory experiences build muscle tone and curiosity all at once. Bath time becomes less about getting clean and more about exploring what it means to *feel*, to play, to move in a different world.

If the weather's kind, bring the play outdoors. A blanket in the park introduces a tapestry of new sensations, the rustle of leaves, the scent of grass, the flutter of a bird's wings above. Here, tummy time expands into a multisensory adventure, where nature becomes your baby's first teacher.

Each reach, each roll, each giggle is a brick in the foundation of their future. And each shared smile during these sessions deepens the emotional thread between you. This is not just physical growth, it is relational, it is emotional, it is the quiet building of trust.

Language and Communication: A Symphony of Connection

There is something sacred in the way your baby listens to you, those wide, searching eyes, the subtle stillness in their body, as though your voice is the most beautiful thing they've ever heard. And maybe, to them, it is. Your voice is the first poem they know, the first comfort they understand, the first sound of love.

Talking to your baby is not just about teaching them words, it's about showing them the world through your eyes. Every gentle sentence you speak, every silly song you hum while changing a diaper, becomes a building block in their growing mind. You're not just narrating your day, you're laying down neural pathways that will help them one day speak, think, and connect.

Even before they can form words, your baby is communicating. When they coo, gurgle, or squeal, they are sending you signals, trying out the music of their own voice. When you echo those sounds back, you're telling them, *I hear you. I see you. You matter.* That simple exchange is the beginning of conversation, and of feeling truly known.

Don't be afraid to animate your expressions and vary your tone, babies love big emotions and musical inflection. It keeps them engaged and helps them tune into the rhythm of language. Sing lullabies, recite nursery rhymes, tell stories with rising crescendos and hushed pauses. Your baby doesn't need perfect pitch or polished grammar, just the genuine cadence of your love.

Music, again, finds its way into this realm. Songs are stories with melody, and they help little minds hold onto words. Nursery rhymes and lullabies become the early soundtracks of language learning. You might find that your baby smiles or settles faster when a familiar tune begins to play.

If your family speaks more than one language, share them freely and fearlessly. A baby's brain is beautifully adaptable, capable of absorbing multiple languages without confusion. Use books, songs, and everyday conversation to introduce new sounds and phrases. You're not just raising a bilingual child, you're opening their heart to a broader, richer world.

And then there's the sacred ritual of reading aloud. A well-loved board book becomes a bridge between your voice and their imagination. The colors, the rhythm, the gentle turning of pages, it's all an invitation to connect, to cuddle, to dream together. Storytime may start as a quiet moment of bonding, but it will grow into a lifelong love for words and wonder.

The earliest days of parenting are filled with quiet

magic, soft coos, wide-eyed stares, and the wonder of first sounds. In these moments, each word you speak becomes a building block for your baby's understanding of the world. Whether it's a simple conversation as you change a diaper or a lullaby sung in the dim light of evening, you are doing far more than filling the silence. You are nurturing connection. You are teaching the music of language.

Engaging with your baby doesn't require perfection. It's in the silly songs, the animated faces, the gentle commentary of everyday life where the richest learning happens. And then one day, perhaps when you least expect it, they'll echo back a word you've been saying for weeks. Or they'll smile at your familiar tune. Those are the unforgettable moments. Moments when you realize that all those one-sided conversations have been working quietly beneath the surface, creating a foundation for their first real steps into communication.

As you walk this path of parenthood, find comfort in the small things: the babble that fills your kitchen, the soft giggle at your playful rhyme. These are signs that your voice, your love, is shaping how your child will one day speak, think, and understand the world. Every word, every laugh, every lullaby is not only a gift in the moment, but a lasting imprint on their developing mind. So speak freely. Sing without hesitation. These tender exchanges are the heartbeats of early learning and the threads of a bond that will grow stronger with time.

Encouraging Curiosity: Fostering the Spark of Discovery

A baby's curiosity is a beautiful thing, it begins with a glance, a reach, a moment of wonder. Creating an environment that nurtures this natural sense of exploration is like planting seeds of lifelong learning. Through your care, these seeds bloom into confidence, creativity, and joy.

You don't need fancy toys or elaborate setups. A soft rattle, a plush animal, or a colorful stacking ring can become an invitation to explore. These first encounters with sound, shape, and texture build more than play, they build the neural connections that help your baby make sense of their world.

Even a small sensory corner in your home can become a haven of discovery. Crinkly fabrics, bumpy textures, soft and smooth materials, these are simple things, yet they awaken their senses and ignite wonder. Watch their face light up when they discover something new. That spark? That's the beginning of learning, wrapped in the joy of exploration.

Games like peek-a-boo may seem simple, but for a baby, they are magical. Each giggle hides a lesson in how the world works, objects exist even when unseen. It's in these little games that your child begins to understand, to anticipate, to think.

As your baby grows, introduce activities that gently challenge them, stacking cups, simple puzzles, soft books with flaps to lift. Resist the urge to jump in too soon. Give them space to try, to fail, to try again. Your quiet encouragement, your applause, your smile, your words, shows them that effort matters, that they are capable.

Curiosity thrives in freedom. Baby-proofed spaces allow them to explore without fear, to crawl toward the unknown and stretch their boundaries, both physically and mentally. Let them lead playtime sometimes. Follow their gaze, mirror their actions, be present. In doing so, you are saying, "I see you. I trust you. I'm here with you."

Celebrate the small wins like grasping a toy, figuring out how to roll, reaching for something just out of range. These tiny triumphs are huge for them, and your pride becomes their fuel. And don't forget the world outside your walls. A walk in the park, a leaf in their hand, a breeze on their cheeks, nature offers endless sensory invitations that deepen their awareness and ground their learning in beauty.

Repetition is how their world starts to make sense. If they keep returning to the same toy or activity, that's wonderful. Each revisit strengthens what they're learning, giving them the confidence to try the next thing.

Blend fun and learning in ways that feel natural. Puppets, stories, sing-alongs, or just rolling a ball across the floor, these simple joys spark their imagination and support essential growth. Your role isn't to have all the answers, but to stay present in the discovery.

As this chapter closes, take a breath and look at the world through your baby's eyes: full of possibility, color, sound, and warmth. Your presence, your patience, and your love create a world where curiosity feels safe and learning feels like joy. These early days are not just about milestones. They're about moments: shared, celebrated, and savored. And in the next chapter, we'll explore how nurturing emotional connection adds another layer to this rich, beautiful journey of raising a whole-hearted, bright-minded child.

Chapter 8: Overcoming Challenges Together

The Sleep Struggle: Strategies for Better Nights

I remember one night in vivid detail, a night when weariness hung heavy in the air, and every breath felt like an effort. The clock had crept past midnight, and the soft hush of our home was broken only by the steady cries of our newborn. In that fragile silence, I felt the full weight of new parenthood, equal parts overwhelming and deeply, achingly tender.

Sleep struggles are a reality every parent meets face-to-face. It's more than a phase, it's a rite of passage, one that demands patience, tenderness, and the quiet strength that only love can summon. Understanding your baby's unique sleep rhythms can help make those long nights a bit more manageable. Unlike us, babies drift in and out of rest in short bursts, typically 50 to 60 minutes at a time, shifting between deep and light sleep. At first, it may feel confusing and unpredictable, but learning to recognize those subtle signs of tiredness...yawns, eye-rubbing, or fussiness, can help you catch those fleeting windows before they close.

Creating a sleep-nurturing environment can be transformative for everyone in the household. Blackout curtains don't just darken a room, they signal to your baby's body that it's time to rest. A gently humming fan or humidifier can become a soothing backdrop, a familiar sound that helps drown out the rest of the world. And keeping the room cool, between 68 and 72 degrees, can make a world of difference for both comfort and safety. These aren't just small details; they're love in action, the quiet choices that say, *You are safe. You can rest here.*

Equally important is the bedtime ritual, the little sequence of love you repeat each night to gently ease your baby from the energy of the day into the calm of sleep. A warm bath, a soft massage, a slow feeding, a lullaby whispered against their tiny ear, each action becomes a thread in the fabric of security and trust. With time, these patterns begin to speak to your baby in a language deeper than words: *It's time to rest. You're not alone.*

Letting natural light guide your baby during the day, and soft, low lighting take over as evening falls, helps their body learn the rhythm of day and night. As the sun sets and the house quiets, those transitions teach your child, little by little, what it means to slow down and surrender to rest.

And you...you are part of this rhythm too. Sharing the nighttime load isn't just about logistics. It's about preserving your own spirit and supporting each other through the beautiful, chaotic miracle of parenting. Take turns when you can. Speak openly about your limits. Let the love between you grow stronger not just in the joy-filled moments, but in the weary ones too, the ones where a shared yawn and a tired smile say, *We've got this.*

Sleep Log and Reflection: Making Sense of the Nights

Sometimes, clarity comes through reflection. Try keeping a simple sleep log over a few weeks. Record when your baby sleeps and wakes, what happened just before, and how long each cycle lasted. You might be surprised by the patterns that emerge, tiny clues that can help fine-tune your routine and offer both of you more rest.

Take note of your own sleep, too. Seeing the full picture, yours and your baby's, can spark practical adjustments. Maybe it's shifting a feeding time, trying a new bedtime ritual, or letting yourself nap when the baby does. The act of observing without judgment can be a powerful way to reclaim a sense of calm in the unknown.

Celebrate the small victories. One longer nap, one smoother bedtime, one less wake-up. These are not just milestones, they're proof of your effort, your care, and your adaptability. Every peaceful night, however rare at first, is a gentle reminder: you're learning this together.

Colic and Crying: Gentle Power in a Father's Hands

There is a sound that cuts through even the deepest stillness, a baby's cry in the night. It stirs something primal in you, a fierce and tender need to comfort. And yet, sometimes, no matter what you do, the crying doesn't stop. It's a helplessness that lingers in your chest, a question without an answer. This might be colic.

Colic is more than just crying. It's relentless, often lasting over three hours, at the same time each day, with your baby curled in discomfort, fists clenched, tiny body taut with distress. It's hard to watch. It's even harder to soothe. But knowing what it is can help. And knowing you're not alone can make all the difference.

This is where the "5 S's" come in, simple, time-tested techniques that echo the safety of the womb:

- **Swaddling** offers the snugness they once knew.
- **Side or stomach holding** shifts pressure and soothes.
- **Shushing** mimics your heartbeat's rhythm.
- **Swinging** recreates gentle motion.
- **Sucking** through a pacifier or feeding brings comfort.

These aren't just tricks, they're love translated into action. Your baby may not yet understand your words, but they feel your steady arms, your soft voice, your quiet determination to help them feel okay again.

Other methods, like baby-wearing or gentle tummy massages, can help both of you. Wearing your baby close against your chest not only calms their cries with warmth and rhythm but allows you to stay connected while tending to the world around you. You become their safe haven, their quiet anchor in the storm.

And it's okay to feel overwhelmed. It's okay to cry, too. This isn't about getting it perfect. It's about showing up, night after night, with a heart full of love and arms ready to hold.

There are moments in parenthood when your heart aches in sync with your baby's cries. Their tiny body twists in discomfort, fists clenched, legs drawn to their belly, and you would trade anything to take away their pain. In these moments, gently massaging your baby's tummy in slow, clockwise circles can offer a small but powerful comfort, especially if gas or digestion issues are the culprit. It's a humble act, but one filled with care, a way to tell your baby, without words, *I'm here, and I'm trying.*

Still, amidst all your efforts to soothe, it's just as important to turn inward and care for yourself. When the crying stretches on and nothing seems to work, stress can mount fast. Your breath quickens, your body tenses, and the helplessness creeps in. But your calm is your baby's anchor. Practicing something as simple as deep breathing can help you reclaim it. Inhale slowly through your nose, exhale gently through your mouth. Let each breath remind you that you're doing your best, and that's enough.

There is no shame in needing a pause. If the moment overwhelms you, place your baby gently in a safe space and give yourself a few minutes to reset. Step outside, splash water on your face, or simply sit in silence. These brief breaks aren't failures, they're lifelines. Reach out to your partner or a loved one. Let them take over for a bit. Your well-being matters too.

The Power of Partnership in Colic Moments

When colic enters your world, it doesn't just affect your baby, it tests every ounce of your emotional and physical energy as a parent. That's why leaning on your partner is not only helpful but essential. Keep talking. Share what worked and what didn't. Try new methods together. Trade off responsibilities, and more importantly, check in on each other's mental and emotional state.

Teamwork here is about more than just "taking turns", it's about seeing each other's fatigue and stepping in with empathy. It's saying, *I know this is hard for you too,* and creating space for each of you to rest, reflect, and feel supported. Your baby feels the strength of your unity, even if they can't yet understand it.

Reflection Section: Your Soothing Journal

Keep a journal close. Write down what you try, what soothes your baby, even what doesn't. Over time, you'll begin to see patterns, little clues about what comforts them best. This journal isn't just a log; it's a quiet roadmap of love and trial. Each page is proof of your devotion, your patience, and your growing understanding of your baby's unique rhythms.

Remember: every cry responded to, every gentle touch offered, and every moment endured in the quiet ache of the night, ties the unspoken language of trust between you and your baby.

Tuning Out the Noise: Trusting Yourself Amid Unwanted Advice

Becoming a parent invites a torrent of voices. They arrive with the best intentions, neighbors, relatives, strangers in the checkout line, each offering their two cents on what *you should do.* The flood can be overwhelming. Some advice might be helpful. But much of it? Uninvited noise.

Comments like, "When my kids were babies, we always did this..." are often rooted in love, but they don't always reflect your child's reality, or your parenting style. A simple "Thanks, I'll keep that in mind" is a gracious way to acknowledge them without feeling pressured to follow.

What matters most is your confidence in your own instincts. You *know* your child in ways no one else can. Take time to reflect on the kind of parent you want to be. Do you value raising an empathetic child? A curious one? A resilient one? These values become your compass, guiding your decisions when the outside noise gets too loud.

Celebrate your wins, even the tiny ones. Managing a fussy bedtime, calming a mid-morning meltdown, or just making it through a tough day with grace, these are victories. Let them remind you that you are growing into your role as a parent. You don't have to be perfect. You only have to be present.

Setting Boundaries with Love

When advice turns pushy, don't be afraid to set kind but clear boundaries. If Aunt Susan insists on her way being *the* way, a simple, respectful "I appreciate your thoughts, but we're doing what feels right for our family" can defuse tension without inviting further debate.

These moments are not about confrontation; they're about protecting your space as a parent. Redirect the conversation to lighter topics or shared memories. Maintain connection without compromising your confidence.

Finding Support That Resonates

In a world flooded with opinions, choose wisely whom you listen to. Lean on your pediatrician or trusted parenting resources. Join online or in-person communities focused on evidence-based practices and emotional support. These spaces aren't about judgment, they're about shared growth, offering comfort in knowing you're not alone in the struggle.

Reflection Section: Defining Your Parenting Values

Take five quiet minutes and jot down the values that matter most to you as a parent. Write what you want your child to remember you for, not what others expect, but what you *believe in.* Revisit these notes when doubt creeps in. They'll be your anchor, your reminder that you're leading with intention and love.

At the end of the day, your parenting path is yours alone to walk. You're not failing when you question, stumble, or feel unsure, you're learning. Every choice you make, every moment you push through the exhaustion, every time you trust your gut, you are building something deeply meaningful: a bond with your child built on love, intention, and presence. That's more powerful than any advice could ever be.

The Art of Compromise: Working Through Parenting Disagreements

Parenting often feels like an intimate, improvised dance, sometimes graceful, sometimes clumsy, always requiring awareness, rhythm, and compassion. You move in tandem, sometimes stepping on each other's toes, but with each misstep comes an opportunity to realign. The first and most important step in this dance is acknowledging that no two people parent exactly the same. One of you may flow with spontaneity and gut instincts, while the other leans on schedules and structure. These differences are not flaws; they are expressions of care shaped by personal histories, fears, and hopes.

Recognizing and respecting these differences is how harmony begins. Set aside quiet time together to talk, not about rules or routines, but about values. What do you want your child to grow into? Kindness? Resilience? Creativity? These conversations are less about logistics and more about dreams. And when parenting styles clash, come back to this shared foundation. You are not opponents trying to win a debate, you are partners trying to raise a human being together.

Effective communication becomes the bridge between your differences. Words matter, especially when feelings are raw. Saying, "I feel invisible during the bedtime rush," invites empathy, while "You never help" builds walls. Shifting from blame to vulnerability opens the door to being seen and heard. And don't just listen, truly listen. Put down the phone, make eye contact, nod, repeat back what you hear: "So you're feeling stretched thin during weekends, and you need us to plan them more intentionally?" These small gestures carry enormous emotional weight. They say, "You matter to me."

Inevitably, there will be moments when emotions flare and words stumble out faster than hearts can catch up. In those moments, step back...not away. Take a breath, take a walk, come back when the fire has softened. Conflict is not failure; it's a signal that something inside you needs tenderness, and so does your partner. The goal isn't to win, it's to understand. Compromise is not about letting go of what you hold dear. It's about finding a middle place where love speaks louder than pride. Maybe that looks like alternating bedtime duties, or letting one parent take the lead in the morning while the other resets. Maybe it's simply agreeing to try something different, together. When both voices are heard, solutions stop being sacrifices and start becoming shared commitments.

Presenting a united front doesn't mean you always agree, it means your child sees stability, even when you're working through disagreement behind the scenes. Kids feel everything. When they witness kindness between their parents, when they see the gentle act of one backing the other, they feel safe. That's what matters most. They don't need perfect parents, they need connected ones.

This process of learning how to parent together is one of the most intimate acts of love. It's how you grow not just as caregivers, but as partners, trusting each other more deeply with every challenge weathered and every triumph shared.

So when it feels hard, and it will, remember that every misstep is just another part of the dance. You are not alone on the floor. You are in this together, learning the rhythm of parenting, step by loving step.

Reflection Prompt: Core Values Check-In

Take time to each jot down three values you want your child to embody. Then share them aloud. Where do they overlap? Where do they differ? Use this as a foundation for future decisions, knowing you're building a home where both your hearts are heard.

Chapter 9: Building a Strong Parenting Partnership

Co-Parenting Principles: Cultivating Equality at Home

I first glimpsed the quiet strength of true partnership in the midst of life's ordinary chaos, during a particularly frantic dinner prep. My wife, cradling our lively newborn in one arm, moved with a calm grace while I maneuvered around the stove, dicing vegetables with theatrical urgency, trying not to burn the stew. Our eyes met over the clatter of pots and the baby's delighted squeals, and in that fleeting moment, an unspoken accord passed between us. We were teammates in the fullest sense, shouldering the weight of parenthood together, each step guided by mutual trust, respect, and shared purpose. This chapter is an invitation to explore the essence of co-parenting: a partnership defined not by perfection, but by a deep commitment to equality, empathy, and unity.

At its core, equality in parenting does not mean splitting tasks down the middle or mirroring one another's roles. Instead, it means honoring each parent's distinct strengths and leaning into them with intention. Perhaps one of you has a natural instinct for calming tantrums, while the other navigates the intricacies of pediatric schedules with practiced ease. Recognizing these differences isn't a weakness, it's the foundation of a powerful alliance. Through open conversation and reflection, each partner's contributions can be seen, appreciated, and celebrated. It's in this recognition that true balance is born, one that supports both partners and enriches the home with a sense of fairness and unity.

A key pillar of co-parenting is **shared decision-making**. Whether choosing your baby's first foods or mapping out the future of their education, involving both parents in these decisions reinforces the idea that your child's wellbeing is a joint endeavor. Shared choices diffuse potential resentment, foster ownership, and ensure that both voices are heard and valued. Through open, consistent communication, decisions become less about compromise and more about collaboration, an evolving dialogue that deepens trust and unites your visions for your family's future. Of course, juggling professional demands with domestic responsibilities is no easy feat. One gentle yet effective solution is a **rotating chore chart**, a simple visual reminder that the home is a shared space built by shared effort. When tasks are regularly rotated, empathy naturally grows, each partner experiences the full spectrum of responsibilities and learns to value the other's work. Additionally, advocating for flexible work arrangements is an essential aspect of co-parenting equality. Conversations with employers about accommodating family needs can create the space necessary to show up fully, both at home and in the workplace.

Just as children grow and change, so too must your

co-parenting rhythms. Schedule regular check-ins or monthly family meetings to evaluate what's working, what isn't, and what needs shifting. These gatherings provide a safe space for honest feedback and gentle realignment, preventing stagnation and allowing your dynamic to evolve alongside your family's needs. It's in these quiet recalibrations that your partnership deepens, as each partner feels seen, heard, and supported.

Visual Element: Co-Parenting Chore Chart

Make the chore chart a family creation: colorful, fun, and fluid. Use bright markers, stickers, or themed visuals to assign tasks, turning it into an enjoyable and meaningful ritual. Rotate responsibilities weekly to foster a deeper appreciation for each other's efforts, and keep the spirit light, this is a shared life, not a ledger of labor.

In building a home rooted in co-parenting principles, you're not only nurturing your bond as partners but also modeling healthy relationships for your child. When children witness fairness, mutual respect, and open communication between their caregivers, they absorb those values as their own. They learn, not through instruction, but through observation, watching the small, consistent acts of love that form the bedrock of a stable, nurturing home.

Conflict Resolution: Meeting Disagreements with Grace

Even in the most harmonious households, conflict is inevitable, especially in the whirlwind of early parenthood. One moment you're debating bedtime songs, and the next, you're unraveling deep philosophical differences on child-rearing. Often, these tensions stem from core beliefs: one parent may favor structured routines, while the other leans toward a more flexible, intuitive approach. Add to that the pressures of sleepless nights, financial worries, and shifting identities, and small misunderstandings can quickly escalate into larger emotional storms.

But conflict, when approached with grace and understanding, can become a tool for growth rather than a source of division. The first step is **active listening**, truly hearing your partner without interruption or defensiveness. When one speaks and the other listens with presence and empathy, a new kind of conversation emerges, one grounded not in who's right, but in what matters. Taking a pause during heated exchanges can help both partners return with clearer minds and softer hearts, reducing the risk of saying things they'll later regret.

Creating a set of **conflict ground rules** is a powerful way to keep disagreements respectful and productive. Agree never to attack character, focus instead on behaviors and solutions. Choose your timing wisely, and prioritize privacy; resolving issues away from children protects their emotional safety and reinforces a respectful household culture. These rules don't restrict you, they liberate you, providing structure that transforms discord into constructive dialogue.

When viewed with perspective, conflict reveals what each person values most. After the dust settles, take time to reflect, not to assign blame, but to understand what the disagreement uncovered about your needs and communication styles. Celebrate your victories, however small. Each resolved conflict is proof that your partnership can weather storms, and emerge stronger. These are not just disputes to overcome, but milestones of maturity that signal your growth as a team.

In learning to navigate conflict with kindness and clarity, you teach your child perhaps the most enduring lesson of all: love is not the absence of disagreement, but the choice to keep showing up for one another, even when it's hard.

Exercise: Conflict Reflection Journal

Consider keeping a *Conflict Reflection Journal*, a quiet space where you can thoughtfully record moments of disagreement, how they were resolved, and the wisdom gathered in their wake. Revisiting these experiences allows you to notice patterns: what helped, what hindered, and what could be refined. In doing so, you sharpen your communication and gain a deeper understanding of how your relationship evolves through challenge.

Approaching conflict with grace is a learned skill, requiring patience, humility, and persistence. Yet, the reward is profound. By uncovering the roots of tension, developing respectful ground rules, and viewing disagreements not as setbacks but as opportunities for mutual growth, you cultivate a partnership that is both resilient and nurturing. In this process, your child becomes a quiet observer, learning, through your example, the language of empathy, negotiation, and repair. Every resolved conflict becomes a building block in the architecture of a deeply respectful and loving home.

Celebrating Wins: Recognizing Each Other's Contributions

Amid the hustle of family life, it's easy to overlook the

small, sustaining acts that keep everything moving, refilling the diaper bag, preparing a favorite meal, handling a midnight wake-up. Yet, it is precisely these gestures that deserve acknowledgment. A heartfelt "thank you" carries the power to soften exhaustion and strengthen emotional connection.

Expressing gratitude, especially when it's specific, says, *I see you.* It affirms the everyday efforts that often go unnoticed. Something as simple as, "Thank you for getting up with the baby last night, it gave me the chance to truly rest," not only validates effort but also fosters a culture of care and recognition.

Consider starting a *Gratitude Journal* together. It doesn't need to be elaborate, just a few lines here and there, noting the gestures that made a difference. Whether it's folding laundry or managing playdates, this simple practice becomes a growing archive of mutual appreciation. During more difficult days, it can serve as a reminder of all the invisible ways love shows up.

Elevate this practice further by creating *rituals of appreciation.* Weekly check-ins, perhaps over Saturday morning coffee or a quiet evening once the children are asleep, can become sacred moments of connection. Use these times to reflect on what you've admired in one another that week. These exchanges don't need grandeur, just honesty and warmth. They turn appreciation into a living part of your shared rhythm, helping to ward off resentment and deepen your connection.

Introduce joy and gratitude to the entire family by making a *Gratitude Jar.* Invite everyone, even young children, to drop in small notes of thanks whenever they feel moved. Reading them together later fosters emotional literacy and shows that appreciation is not just spoken, it's shared, felt, and celebrated as a family.

Celebrate growth, too, not just accomplishments, but the subtle evolutions. Perhaps your partner has become more patient, or you've learned to manage stress with greater grace. These milestones, when acknowledged, inspire continued growth and mutual admiration.

Encouraging positive reinforcement also helps maintain motivation in co-parenting. Small rewards for achieving shared goals, like a favorite dessert or an extra hour of rest, signal that effort matters. It's not about the scale of the reward, but the spirit of recognition.

Setting and revisiting shared goals, whether planning a trip or simply reworking the morning routine, reinforces your partnership. These joint pursuits invite collaboration, purpose, and a sense of accomplishment that you both can own. Celebrating each step forward, no matter how modest, infuses your home with purpose and pride.

Ultimately, learning to celebrate wins, big and small, builds a powerful foundation of gratitude. It transforms the everyday into a source of strength, deepens your bond, and creates a nurturing emotional atmosphere where both partners, and children, can thrive.

The Power of Routine: Creating Stability for Your Family

I remember it clearly, an icy morning, the aroma of

coffee curling through the kitchen, our baby murmuring softly after a peaceful night. My wife and I exchanged a quiet smile across the breakfast table. In that moment, our morning routine felt like a warm embrace, a grounding rhythm amid the chaos of new parenthood. What could have been disarray became harmony, thanks to the gentle predictability we had created.

Routines bring not just order, but comfort. Morning and evening rituals shape the flow of your day, making transitions smoother and more peaceful. Children, in particular, thrive on consistency. It helps them feel secure, cared for, and anchored in their world.

As your child grows, so should your routines. What works for a sleepy infant may not suit a curious toddler. Flexibility becomes your ally. An earlier bedtime, more interactive stories, or a choice between two pajamas, these small adjustments allow your routine to grow with your child. Including them in planning instills confidence and decision-making skills early on.

But balance is essential. While routines provide structure, room for spontaneity adds delight. Be open to the unexpected, a surprise visit to the park, a dance party before dinner. These unplanned moments inject joy and remind your family that while rhythm matters, so does flexibility.

And when special occasions arise, holidays, family visits, celebrations, allow your routine to bend. Let bedtime stretch for an extra story or a cozy movie. Such variations teach your children that while routines bring peace, adaptability brings resilience.

In essence, routines are more than habits, they're the

threads that stitch your family life together. They provide a dependable rhythm through the noise of daily life, nurturing both security and togetherness. And in those still moments, be it a shared breakfast or a bedtime cuddle, you'll find not just stability, but joy.

Shared routines are far more than a string of repeated actions, they are threads that quietly stitch together the fabric of family life. Within these familiar patterns, bonds deepen and communication flourishes. Creating simple, meaningful traditions, like a Thursday evening game night or pancakes sizzling on Saturday mornings, invites togetherness and turns the ordinary into memory-making magic. Amid the flurry of daily responsibilities, these rituals offer an anchoring sense of belonging, moments that are eagerly anticipated and fondly remembered.

Beyond togetherness, routines become gentle opportunities for connection. A quick exchange during dinner prep or an unrushed breakfast can blossom into heartfelt conversations. In these seemingly casual moments, family members find the space to express themselves, fostering an environment where voices are heard and emotions are shared.

Though routines may seem mundane on the surface, they offer something profound: a sense of stability, love, and grounding. They tether your family to the present while nurturing the emotional soil from which children grow. More than rigid schedules, routines are adaptable frameworks that flow with your family's natural rhythm, responsive to your evolving needs, yet consistent enough to provide comfort and continuity. As you move forward in this book, carry with you the quiet wisdom of routine. It is in the predictability of these practices that children find security, and within their flexible structure that they learn resilience and independence. The true strength of routine lies not just in order, but in its capacity to draw families closer and support each person's unfolding growth.

In the chapters ahead, we'll explore how to deepen these connections by nurturing emotional bonds, building upon the groundwork laid by shared routines and daily closeness.

Chapter 10:
Embracing Change and Growth

The Growth Mindset: Embracing Change as a Dad

The moment I first held my newborn, something inside me shifted. It felt as though the very ground beneath my feet gave way, and in its place emerged a new world, foreign, unpredictable, and deeply transformative. My identity, once firmly rooted, began to stretch and bend to meet the demands of fatherhood. Everything I thought I knew about myself was quietly rearranged to make space for this extraordinary new chapter.

It is in this continuous transformation that the concept of a *growth mindset* becomes not just helpful, but essential. Introduced by psychologist Carol Dweck, a growth mindset is the belief that our abilities and intelligence are not fixed traits, but qualities that can evolve through effort, curiosity, and resilience. In the ever-changing landscape of parenting, this mindset becomes a vital compass, guiding us not to perfection, but to progress.

In contrast, a fixed mindset assumes our capacities are carved in stone. It views challenges as threats and failure as a verdict. But fatherhood invites a different approach. It asks us to greet every diaper disaster and sleepless night not as obstacles, but as lessons. It offers daily, sometimes hourly, chances to grow in patience, empathy, and resourcefulness.

Adopting a growth mindset as a father means setting

small but intentional goals, perhaps to remain calm during a tantrum, or to discover new ways to connect during play. These goals act as stepping stones, helping you track your evolution as a parent. When challenges arise, like picky eating or bedtime struggles, view them as opportunities to experiment and learn. Trying a new recipe together or crafting a more soothing bedtime ritual transforms frustration into connection.

Your mindset shapes your child's, too. By modeling curiosity, persistence, and optimism, you teach your child that effort matters more than immediate success. Praise becomes more powerful when it recognizes perseverance: *"I saw how you kept trying different pieces until the puzzle was complete. That was really thoughtful of you."* Such affirmations help children internalize the value of growth, giving them confidence to tackle the unknown.

Encourage exploration by introducing your child to new experiences, whether it's watching ants in the backyard or wandering through a science museum. These moments spark imagination, encourage questions, and teach them to approach life with open, eager minds. Curiosity becomes their lifelong guide, teaching them that the world is vast, fascinating, and theirs to discover.

And when things go wrong, and they will, resist the urge to see it as failure. If bedtime becomes a nightly battle, consider it a prompt for adjustment, not defeat. Perhaps a new story, a calming playlist, or an earlier wind-down time will make a difference. Look to books, friends, or your own intuition for ideas. A growth mindset reminds us that each day is a fresh slate, a new chance to learn, pivot, and try again.

Fatherhood, like all meaningful growth, is not a straight line. It is a series of moments, some tender, some testing, all carrying within them the potential to transform you into a wiser, more present version of yourself. Embrace the changes. Lean into the learning. And remember: every effort you make is a gift, not only to your child, but to the man you are becoming.

Reflection Section: The Growth Mindset Journal

Begin a "Growth Mindset Journal" as a personal companion to your parenting journey, a space to explore challenges, document your evolving strategies, and celebrate growth. Use it to reflect on what worked, what could be refined, and the wisdom gained along the way. This journal becomes more than a record; it transforms into a reservoir of resilience and a quiet reminder of how far you've come. In times of doubt or discouragement, its pages offer encouragement. In moments of triumph, they hold your legacy of perseverance and progress.

Fatherhood is not a destination but a lifelong transformation, an unfolding story of lessons, love, and growth. Embracing a growth mindset not only elevates your experience as a parent, but also lays the groundwork for a home where change is welcomed, learning is habitual, and evolving together becomes a family tradition.

Learning from Mistakes: The Path to Better Parenting

Mistakes are not detours, they are the path itself. They are part of every parent's story: forgetting the diaper bag, misjudging nap time, overreacting when patience runs thin. These moments may feel like failures, but they are in fact vital markers along the road to wisdom. Embracing them with grace and humility fosters a home where imperfection is accepted, and growth is inevitable.

To truly grow, we must not merely acknowledge our mistakes, but understand them. Reflecting constructively, perhaps in your journal, enables you to see patterns, uncover insights, and adjust your approach. Open communication with your partner can further illuminate alternative strategies and strengthen your shared parenting foundation. These honest conversations create cohesion, aligning your efforts and deepening the bond between you.

Once insights are gleaned, take action. Transform past missteps into meaningful change. If bedtime has become a battleground, introduce calming rituals or modify routines to create a gentler transition. These adjustments show your children that learning never stops, and that every challenge is an opportunity to improve.

Modeling this process for your children teaches them a powerful lesson: that mistakes do not define us, they refine us. Share your own experiences, not just your successes. Let them see how you navigated setbacks, what you learned, and how you grew. Encourage them to reflect with questions like, "What did this teach you?" or "What could we try next time?" These conversations nurture critical thinking and inner strength, arming them with the tools to face life's hurdles with grace.

Everyday moments hold space for this kind of

learning. A spilled drink can lead to a discussion about coordination. A forgotten homework assignment becomes a chance to talk about planning. These are not just "teachable moments," they're invitations to connect, explore, and evolve together.

By embracing mistakes as fertile ground for growth, you model resilience and compassion. You show your children that life isn't about never falling, but about rising thoughtfully and stronger each time. In the grand journey of fatherhood, every stumble can lead you closer to the parent you aspire to be.

Adapting to Your New Normal: Flexibility in Fatherhood

Fatherhood demands both steadiness and surrender. Life with children is anything but predictable. One moment you're managing the school drop-off seamlessly, and the next, you're navigating a full-scale meltdown in the cereal aisle. The family landscape is always shifting, growing children, evolving relationships, new responsibilities, and to thrive, we must meet this change not with resistance, but with grace.

Like a river adjusting its course around stones, flexibility allows us to flow through the unexpected with resilience. It doesn't mean abandoning structure, but embracing it with elasticity. When plans fall apart, the flexible father pauses, not to panic, but to pivot. He sees detours not as dead ends, but as opportunities to discover something new.

Flexibility is an active practice. Cultivate it by broadening your perspective in challenging moments. Ask, "What else might this situation be showing me?" Let go of the need to control every detail, and instead, cultivate the capacity to respond wisely. Grounding techniques, like mindful breathing or short meditations, can help restore clarity when chaos looms, guiding your reactions from impulse to intention.

Yet, even amidst fluidity, children still crave structure. Routines anchor them. They provide a rhythm to the day, a sense of security in a world that often feels vast and uncertain. The key is in the balance, routines that guide, but bend when needed. If a planned park trip is rained out, turn your living room into a jungle adventure. Let laughter fill the gaps left by thwarted plans.

Flexibility in fatherhood doesn't mean always having the perfect response. It means showing up with openness, curiosity, and love. It means understanding that adaptation is not weakness, it's wisdom in motion. When your children see you adjust without losing your center, they learn to do the same. They learn that home is not a rigid place, but a living, breathing space where change is not feared but embraced.

And in that flexible, forgiving space, family flourishes. Life's major shifts, welcoming a new child or moving to a new home, can stir a whirlwind of emotions. Yet with flexibility, these transitions can become smoother, more meaningful chapters in your family's story. True preparation extends beyond logistics; it includes emotional readiness and clear communication. Encourage open conversations with your family about upcoming changes. Invite each voice, no matter how small, to be heard. This openness fosters connection and helps set realistic expectations, turning uncertainty into a shared adventure where everyone feels respected and supported.

Growth also comes from listening to others who've walked similar paths. Reach out to fellow parents. Share experiences, swap strategies, and find comfort in knowing you're not navigating this alone. A community of parents, all striving, adapting, and learning together, is a powerful reminder that flexibility does not mean disorder. Instead, it's about embracing change with grace, understanding that plans will shift, children will grow in unpredictable ways, and life will continue to test and refine your patience. Flexibility becomes the bridge between life's unexpected turns and your family's steady heartbeat. Think of adaptability as a personalized toolkit, filled with creative approaches for any curveball life throws your way. It's being resourceful during a hectic bedtime or finding delight in impromptu solutions on long drives. Adaptability threads together the fabric of your family life, stitching joy and strength into both the planned and the spontaneous.

In times of transformation, flexibility becomes your compass, not just to endure, but to flourish together. Challenges then become opportunities for unity and growth, strengthening your role as a father and partner. Embrace the evolution of your family's story with openness, knowing that each new chapter offers deeper understanding, more affection, and a legacy built on shared strength. Let flexibility guide you through the unpredictable beauty of fatherhood, nurturing a home alive with connection, laughter, and love.

Cultivating Patience: The Quiet Power Within

Though patience may not be the first trait associated with fatherhood, it is undoubtedly one of its most vital. The day-to-day realities of parenting, spilled cereal, sudden meltdowns, marathon bedtime negotiations, can fray even the calmest nerves. But in these very moments, patience emerges as your quiet superpower, transforming chaos into connection and pressure into presence.

Patience isn't a trait you're simply born with, it's a skill, one strengthened through awareness and practice. Begin by recognizing what triggers your impatience. Whether it's the rush of the morning routine or the strain of a child's outburst, awareness is the first step toward mastery. With this insight, you can shift from reacting to responding, from frustration to empathy.

Mindfulness can be a powerful ally here. Simple techniques like deep breathing or a few minutes of daily meditation can help anchor your mind. In the thick of a tough moment, your baby crying inconsolably or your toddler refusing to cooperate, a few centered breaths can reset your emotional state, allowing you to respond with calm instead of combativeness. These practices build the kind of resilience that transforms stress into a source of strength.

Practicing patience is not about silence, it's about presence. When your child refuses to share or acts out, pause. Breathe. Then offer gentle guidance rather than swift correction. Your calm becomes their model. In doing so, you're not only resolving conflict but showing them what emotional regulation and

122

respectful dialogue look like.

Teach patience by living it. Let your children witness you navigating life's small delays with composure, waiting in lines, managing changes in plans, or calmly dealing with disruptions. Invite them into activities that require waiting and taking turns, puzzles, board games, planting seeds. These moments imprint a quiet message: patience brings reward, and delay can deepen delight.

Stories can also serve as powerful teachers. Share tales, real or imagined, of individuals who achieved great things through persistent patience. These stories give patience a face, a narrative, a purpose. They help children see it not as a restriction but as a virtue that paves the path to wisdom, success, and peace.

Within your home, cultivate an atmosphere where patience is both practiced and praised. Let it infuse your daily rhythms, your conversations, your corrections, and your celebrations. Your children, attuned to your energy, will absorb this as part of their own character, learning to approach life with understanding rather than urgency.

As we close this chapter on embracing change, remember: patience is not about passive waiting. It's about how you carry yourself through each moment. It's a posture of grace, an offering of understanding, a bridge to connection. With every patient response, you nourish the emotional soil in which your children grow resilient, secure, and kind.

And now, with patience and flexibility guiding your path, you are ready to explore how these virtues shape the traditions and memories that define your family.

Together, they become the foundation of a legacy built on love, strength, and enduring joy.

Chapter 11
Cultivating Community and Connection

Finding Your Tribe: Dads' Groups and Networks

I'll never forget the first time I stepped into a room full of other dads. My heart pounded like a drum in my chest, nerves crackling with questions: *Would I fit in? Would they understand me?* I felt exposed, like I was walking into a spotlight with no script. But as the evening unfolded, something beautiful happened. I saw myself in these men. They weren't perfect. They were raw, real, fumbling through fatherhood just like me, craving connection, aching to be seen, and desperate to know they weren't alone. That night shifted something deep inside me. I realized that finding your tribe as a father isn't a luxury, it's a lifeline.

Joining a dads' group isn't just about trading potty-training hacks or venting about sleepless nights. It's about anchoring yourself to a support system that sees you, hears you, and lifts you when you can't stand on your own. It's about being part of something that reminds you: *You don't have to do this alone.*

Finding the right group is a personal journey, like trying on shoes until one fits just right. It has to feel natural. Aligned with your values. Safe. Begin by exploring community centers, local bulletin boards, or parenting-focused social media groups. If showing up in person isn't doable, don't hesitate to look online. Virtual dads' communities offer flexibility and can be just as powerful. There's something incredible about hearing another dad from halfway around the world say, *"I get it."* That kind of connection crosses time zones, and breaks down emotional walls.

Why It Matters

When you open yourself up to other fathers, you tap into something profoundly human: shared struggle and shared strength. You realize you're not broken, you're just human. You're not failing, you're learning. The power of hearing someone say, *"Me too,"* cannot be overstated. It's validation. It's healing. And sometimes, it's exactly what keeps you going when everything feels overwhelming.

These groups also offer new ways of thinking. One dad's bedtime strategy might change your entire evening routine. Another's way of handling tantrums might make your home feel a little more peaceful. Together, we collect wisdom and courage, not from experts, but from one another.

And then, without even realizing it, some of these dads stop being just group members. They become brothers. You laugh together. Share milestones. Cry when it's hard. Celebrate each other's wins like they're your own. Whether it's grabbing coffee, organizing a playdate, or just checking in after a rough week, these moments form the kind of friendship that sustains you, not just as a parent, but as a person.

Becoming Part of the Group

Being in a group isn't about blending in, it's about showing up. Your story matters. Your voice adds to the chorus. Speak up. Listen deeply. Share openly.

Respect differences, because every father's path is different. Embrace that diversity, it makes the group richer. And if you feel called to do more, take on a role: lead a discussion, coordinate an event, or mentor someone who's new. You'll grow in ways you never expected.

Simple Ways to Make the Most of It

Bring a mental checklist to your next gathering, nothing fancy, just a few stories, questions, or thoughts you're willing to share. Think about how you want to show up. And remember, some of the most powerful connections happen not when you're speaking, but when you're listening...really listening. Ask questions like, *"How did that feel for you?"* or *"What helped you get through that?"* These conversations aren't just informative, they're transformative.

Interactive Tool: The Dad Group Discovery Guide

Create your own "Dad Group Discovery Guide." Write down what matters to you, your values, your interests, what you need emotionally and practically from a group. Then share it with your partner or loved ones and ask for their input. You'll gain fresh insight into what kind of community will truly feed your spirit. This is more than just joining a group, it's choosing a space that reflects the kind of father you want to be.

The Gift of Vulnerability

One of the most life-changing moments in my journey as a dad was the first time I let my guard down. I spoke, really spoke, about the fear I felt. The anger. The guilt. The exhaustion. I expected silence or judgment. Instead, I was met with nods. With tears. With *"I've been there too."* That moment taught me that vulnerability isn't weakness, it's power. It takes real strength to say, *"I don't have all the answers."* And when we do, we give others permission to be real too.

Creating a safe space for these kinds of conversations is sacred work. Set clear expectations for respect and confidentiality. Make room for all voices. And always, always lead with empathy. This is how we build something that lasts. Something that heals. Something that matters.

Finding your tribe isn't about fixing yourself, it's about finding people who remind you you're already enough. Who meet you where you are and walk with you as you grow. These dads become your anchor, your mirror, and your cheerleaders. They see you in your darkest hours and your proudest moments. And in the process, they become something more than friends, they become family.

So step into that room. Send that message. Join that call. Let the walls come down. Because in the vulnerability, in the stories, in the shared silence and the laughter, you just might find yourself.

And you'll know: *You've found your tribe.*

The impact of storytelling on personal growth is profound and far-reaching. When you take the time to share your own story, you naturally enter a state of self-reflection. This reflective process often unveils insights that might otherwise remain buried beneath the surface of daily life. As you recount your experiences, you begin to recognize moments of growth, patterns of behavior, and areas where change or healing might still be needed. Telling your story isn't just about the past, it's about gaining clarity on who you are now and who you're becoming. At the same time, listening to the stories of others broadens your perspective. Hearing how another father navigated a similar challenge or overcame a different kind of struggle can challenge assumptions and inspire new ways of thinking. This mutual exchange of narratives forms a powerful foundation for personal transformation, allowing you to reevaluate your own approach to parenting in a space where continuous growth is not just encouraged but expected.

Vulnerability lies at the heart of this process. When one father opens up about his fears, doubts, or missteps, it creates a ripple effect that makes it safer for others to do the same. By responding with encouragement, empathy, and genuine interest, the community grows stronger and more connected. Sharing stories of vulnerability fosters trust and builds an environment where openness is not only welcomed but becomes a shared norm. In this space, emotional honesty is no longer the exception, it becomes part of the community's culture. This kind of supportive atmosphere is essential for forming deeper relationships and forging meaningful bonds between fathers who might otherwise feel isolated in their experiences. Vulnerability doesn't weaken a group; it fortifies it. Each story shared and received with kindness becomes a building block for a stronger, more resilient fatherhood collective.

Techniques for Comfortable Storytelling

To make storytelling more accessible and less intimidating, it helps to create environments where sharing becomes a natural part of group interactions. Starting with lighthearted or humorous stories can ease everyone into the habit of opening up, especially when trust is still being built. As comfort grows within the group, deeper and more personal experiences tend to emerge organically. Facilitating this kind of sharing often begins with asking open-ended questions that invite reflection without pressure. Practicing active listening, where each speaker feels heard and valued without judgment, further encourages openness. Simple practices, such as taking turns sharing a recent parenting win or a lesson learned the hard way, can build a consistent routine of honest communication. Over time, storytelling becomes more than a tool, it becomes the thread that weaves the community together, fostering shared learning and collective growth.

As you become more seasoned in your role as a father, it's natural to want to give back. Supporting newer dads is one of the most impactful ways to do this. You don't need to be perfect or have all the answers; your value lies in your lived experience. Offering guidance, practical tips, or even just a listening ear can be deeply reassuring to someone who is navigating the unfamiliar terrain of fatherhood. What may seem like a small gesture to you, sharing how you handled sleepless nights or how you coped with work-life balance, can be exactly the insight someone else needs to hear. Mentorship is not about lecturing; it's about walking alongside someone else, offering support where needed, and reminding them that they are not alone in their journey.

Organizing community-centered activities can further enrich the support network available to new fathers. Hosting workshops or informal Q&A sessions gives dads the chance to learn from one another in a space where curiosity is welcomed and experiences are exchanged freely. Social gatherings, like park meetups or group breakfasts, offer relaxed opportunities for bonding and friendship-building. These events can become lifelines for new dads, helping them form connections and gather insights in a nonjudgmental atmosphere. They also create space for seasoned dads to share time-tested strategies and common pitfalls, equipping newer fathers with tools and confidence as they build their own parenting paths. Each shared experience strengthens the collective wisdom of the group and helps shape a culture of inclusivity, mentorship, and ongoing support.

Beyond the immediate community, volunteering with parenting organizations offers another powerful way to extend your impact. Participating in local support groups or nonprofit initiatives allows you to contribute to programs that uplift fathers and families on a broader scale. Whether it's helping organize events, offering peer support, or contributing to resource materials, your involvement helps shape a landscape where fatherhood is supported and celebrated. Contributing to online forums or digital platforms expands your reach even further, providing guidance and encouragement to dads who may not have access to local communities. By championing inclusive and equitable fatherhood initiatives, you not only help individuals, you contribute to a cultural shift that values and supports engaged parenting for all.

Giving Back: Supporting Newer Dads on Their Journey

The benefits of giving back extend beyond the individuals you help. Offering your time, attention, and care enriches your own life in ways that are both emotional and lasting. It creates a cycle of gratitude and reciprocity where support flows in all directions. When you witness the positive changes your involvement brings, whether it's a newfound confidence in a new dad or the blossoming of friendships within the community, you are reminded of the value of connection and collective strength. These acts of kindness help build resilient, caring fatherhood communities, and their impact often reaches far beyond the moment. They lay the foundation for future generations to understand that support, empathy, and mutual care are not luxuries, they're essential components of a thriving family and community life.

Visual Element: Giving Back Checklist

One way to stay engaged and purposeful in your contributions is to create a personal checklist of ways to give back. This might include opportunities to mentor, volunteer, or organize community events. Updating this list regularly helps you stay aligned with the evolving needs of the fatherhood community and ensures that your efforts remain impactful. In doing so, you reinforce your commitment to fostering connection and growth within the community. Each action, no matter how small, becomes a thread in a larger network of support and transformation.

By stepping into the role of mentor, volunteer, or advocate, you become part of something much larger than yourself. You help to shape a community that prioritizes understanding, connection, and collective growth. You contribute to a world where every dad, no matter his background or experience, feels equipped and supported in his parenting journey. These shared efforts make a tangible difference, not only in individual lives but in the broader culture of fatherhood.

Building a Family Legacy: What You Want to Pass On

Building a family legacy is perhaps the most profound expression of fatherhood. It extends beyond financial inheritance or family heirlooms and touches on the enduring values and principles that shape the lives of your children and grandchildren. As a father, you have the unique opportunity to define what truly matters to you and ensure that those beliefs are passed on. Reflecting on the qualities you want to instill, such as empathy, honesty, resilience, and responsibility, can help ground your family's moral foundation. These values gain deeper meaning when they are discussed openly with your loved ones. Conversations around the dinner table or during quiet evenings at home become meaningful moments where your family begins to understand and embrace a shared set of guiding beliefs.

Creating traditions rooted in those values helps anchor them in daily life. Whether it's a Sunday night family meal, an annual camping trip, or a shared holiday ritual, these traditions become more than routines, they become living expressions of your family's identity. Including cultural, spiritual, or ancestral practices deepens the sense of belonging and connects younger generations to their roots. Traditions provide comfort in uncertain times and create joyful memories that transcend the present. Over time, they grow into cherished touchstones that bind your family across generations.

Recording and sharing family stories can further preserve this legacy. Whether you're writing in a family journal, collecting photo albums, or recording audio memories, these efforts create a rich archive of shared history. These stories capture the laughter, the lessons, and the love that define your family's unique journey. When children grow up hearing these stories, of challenges overcome, values upheld, and dreams pursued, they gain a stronger sense of identity and belonging. These narratives don't just preserve the past; they help shape the future by giving each generation a foundation to build upon.

Instilling a legacy of kindness and contribution is about more than just telling your children to do good, it's about showing them how. When your family engages in community service or volunteer work together, you model empathy and active citizenship. Whether it's helping at a local food bank, organizing a clothing drive, or simply checking in on a neighbor, these shared acts of giving leave an indelible mark on your children's hearts. They grow up understanding that compassion is not a rare virtue but a way of life. These lived lessons will carry forward in their actions, shaping not only who they become but the kind of legacy they, too, will one day leave behind.

In embracing storytelling, supporting others, and intentionally shaping your legacy, you become more than just a father, you become a cornerstone of connection, learning, and love. These acts of presence and purpose ripple outward, influencing not just your family, but your community and future generations. Through your stories, your service, and your values, you help build a world where fatherhood is deeply respected, richly supported, and full of possibility.

Chapter 12: Looking Forward – The Long-Term Dad

There is a quiet moment that comes to every father, the realization that time is both fleeting and expansive. One day, you are chasing your toddler around the kitchen island, and the next, you're watching them pack for college. These transitions remind us that fatherhood is not a phase but a lifelong role, one that evolves with time and calls for new skills, deeper awareness, and unwavering presence. Looking ahead to the future as a long-term dad means embracing this continuous transformation with intention, humility, and hope.

As your child grows, so too must your approach to fatherhood. What once required physical energy and constant oversight gradually gives way to emotional availability, mentorship, and respectful guidance. The long-term dad understands that parenting is not about control but about influence, about planting values that will take root and grow independently. He is no longer the commander of daily routines but the architect of enduring trust. This shift is not always easy. It demands a letting go of what once was, a redefining of what it means to protect, teach, and love. Envisioning the years ahead requires reflection on what kind of man you want your children to see when they look at you as adults. Will they see someone who listened? Someone who admitted when he was wrong, who adapted, who stayed curious about their evolving needs and dreams? Will they remember a dad who made space for them to become who they are, not who he hoped they would be? These are the questions that guide the long-term father. They shape the decisions he makes today and the legacy he hopes to leave tomorrow.

Part of this vision involves preparing for your child's eventual independence. It is one of the greatest paradoxes of parenthood, that success is measured by how well your child can thrive without you. That knowledge should not create distance but rather a deeper motivation to build a foundation strong enough to support that freedom. It means teaching them to think critically, to manage failure, to care for others, and to speak up for themselves. These are the qualities that will serve them when you are no longer by their side.

As children mature, their understanding of the world becomes more nuanced, and so should our conversations with them. The long-term dad doesn't shy away from difficult topics. He is willing to discuss mental health, identity, injustice, love, loss, and purpose, not with lectures, but with openness and mutual respect. He understands that these moments of honesty are what solidify a lifetime bond. They are what transform a parent-child relationship into a lifelong friendship built on truth and trust.

At the same time, it's important to honor your own growth. Being a long-term dad is not just about guiding your child, it's about evolving yourself. Your dreams, too, deserve tending. Whether it's pursuing a creative endeavor, changing careers, building healthier habits, or deepening your own relationships, your personal growth becomes a living example for your children. They watch how you navigate disappointment, how you find joy, how you treat others. They learn from how you carry your burdens and celebrate your victories.

This chapter of fatherhood also invites you to think about what you'll leave behind, not in terms of money or property, but in terms of meaning. Your words, your actions, your presence, these are the things that echo across generations. A long-term dad sees legacy not as a destination but as a continuous act of love. He recognizes that his influence will live in the way his children treat others, in the way they show up for themselves and their communities, in the way they love their own children one day.

Looking forward also means embracing change within the family dynamic. Roles shift as children grow, partners age, and life throws its unpredictable twists. Illness, loss, relocation, career changes, these events call for resilience, adaptability, and grace. The long-term dad anchors himself in the values his family has built together, returning to them in times of upheaval. He leads not by having all the answers but by showing up, again and again, with an open heart and a steady hand.

As you imagine the years to come, think about the traditions you want to carry forward. Perhaps it's a weekly dinner, a yearly vacation, or a simple bedtime ritual that continues even as your child grows older. These rituals matter. They become the constants that hold the family together when everything else changes. They are the threads that connect childhood to adulthood, memory to meaning.

And finally, the long-term dad cherishes presence. Not just being in the room but truly being there, with attention, curiosity, and care. He recognizes that time is the most precious currency he can offer, and he spends it wisely. He knows that sometimes, the most profound moments happen in the quiet, the shared silence during a long car ride, the passing glance of understanding, the unexpected laughter during a family meal.

To be a long-term dad is to choose every day to love with intention, to lead with humility, and to grow alongside the family you helped create. It's not about perfection. It's about presence. It's about leaving behind not just a legacy, but a life that meant something deeply to those who knew you best. As you look forward, may you do so with clarity, with courage, and with the conviction that your love, your values, and your presence will shape generations to come.

Continuous Learning: Staying Informed as Your Child Grows

The journey of parenthood is an ever-evolving landscape. Each year brings new challenges, new questions, and new milestones that demand a fresh perspective. For fathers, staying informed isn't simply a best practice, it's an act of love, an intentional effort to remain present and prepared as their children change and grow. Lifelong learning becomes essential, not just for the child's benefit but for the growth of the parent as well.

Understanding your child's developmental stages: emotionally, socially, cognitively, can be a transformative starting point. It helps to know what behaviors are typical at different ages, what struggles to anticipate, and how to respond in ways that encourage confidence, curiosity, and connection. This doesn't mean memorizing charts or obsessing over timelines, but rather staying open to knowledge and insight. Parenting books, child development podcasts, and expert-led articles offer both practical advice and reassurance. They remind you that seeking help isn't weakness, it's wisdom.

Education isn't confined to reading. Attending parenting seminars or workshops, especially those focused on adolescence, emotional regulation, or technology, equips you with tools that go beyond the day-to-day. In these shared spaces, the voice of experience, whether from professionals or fellow parents, can light the way forward. These gatherings are more than informative, they're connective. They offer a place to be seen, heard, and supported by people navigating the same path.

Expanding Your Toolkit: Learning From a Variety of Sources

Beyond formal education, self-directed exploration can deepen your understanding of your child's world. Reading about child psychology, educational theory, or emotional intelligence not only informs how you guide your child, it changes how you listen to them, how you understand their behavior, and how you respond in difficult moments. Staying up to date on emerging educational technologies and global learning trends helps you support your child's unique style of learning and problem-solving in an increasingly complex world.

The parenting journey is also enriched by participation in communities of learners. Online forums and parent groups on social media are full of people sharing wins, asking hard questions, and offering support. You'll find differing perspectives, but also common truths that transcend culture and location: every parent is doing the best they can with what they know. Being part of these conversations keeps you grounded and curious.

Local parenting groups provide something different: a face-to-face connection. Whether it's a monthly meetup or a casual conversation on the playground, these interactions can be surprisingly powerful. Sometimes, just hearing that another parent has faced the same battle with screen time or anxiety is enough to renew your energy and restore your calm.

Learning Through Living: Everyday Moments That Teach

Learning doesn't always come from books or classes; it lives in your everyday life. Your parenting becomes sharper and more intuitive when you reflect on your daily experiences. Every conversation, every mistake, every bedtime struggle or morning success can hold a lesson, if you take the time to see it.

Invite your child into that learning with you. Shared experiences like cooking, gardening, DIY projects, or exploring nature are rich with opportunities for growth. These aren't just bonding moments, they're practical lessons in patience, problem-solving, and creativity. You are not only teaching them life skills, you're modeling the process of learning itself.

Self-reflection is a powerful but often overlooked tool. Taking time at the end of the day to consider what worked well and what could be improved creates a loop of awareness and accountability. It turns parenting from a reactive process into a reflective one, an act of conscious evolution.

Interactive Element: Start a Parenting Reflection Journal

To nurture growth intentionally, consider starting a parenting reflection journal. Spend a few quiet minutes each day jotting down what worked, what felt off, or what surprised you. Over time, patterns will emerge, insights into your parenting habits, your child's behavior, and your emotional responses.

This journal isn't for perfection, it's for presence. You'll begin to notice the subtle shifts in your child's maturity, the slow-building confidence in your decision-making, and the deepening of your bond. Journaling also provides a grounding space during hard phases, proof that growth has happened before and will happen again.

Balancing Independence and Involvement: Evolving Your Role

As children grow older, the parenting role undergoes a subtle but vital shift. Where once you held their hand through every step, now you are asked to step back, gently, patiently, and intentionally. Balancing involvement with the need to foster independence is one of the most challenging aspects of fatherhood.

This begins with observation. Children often show signs of readiness before they have the language to name it. A request to walk to school alone, a newfound interest in cooking dinner without help, or a desire to manage their schedule, these are cues that they are building confidence and capability. Your response matters. When you support these efforts with encouragement instead of fear, you help them trust their own instincts.

Encouraging autonomy isn't about pushing them into adulthood too soon. It's about giving them permission to try, to fail, to try again, with the safety net of your belief in them. Let them make decisions in daily life, like planning a family outing or managing their allowance. These small experiences build their internal compass and show them that their voice matters.

At the same time, staying actively engaged remains essential. Adolescents, in particular, may appear to need less connection, but in truth, they often crave it more deeply, just in different forms. Establishing regular family rituals helps maintain those threads of closeness. Weekly dinners, game nights, or even a shared TV series become moments of togetherness in an increasingly independent world.

Staying Connected Without Hovering

Presence is powerful, but it doesn't need to be overbearing. The long-term father learns the rhythm of quiet support, the art of stepping in without taking over. When your child talks about their passions, ask questions. Celebrate their wins, however small. Attend their events. Show up in ways that matter to them, even when they don't ask for it. This consistent interest signals that your love isn't conditional, it's dependable.

As the parenting dynamic evolves, so too should your approach. You may become more of a coach than a director, offering guidance only when it's sought, allowing room for them to think through problems on their own. Trusting their judgment becomes both an act of faith and a reflection of your parenting.

Shared decision-making also empowers children. Whether it's helping plan a family vacation, redesigning their bedroom, or contributing to grocery choices, involving them in decisions fosters a sense of agency and belonging. They don't just feel heard, they feel respected.

Reflecting on Growth: Yours and Theirs

Parenting, at its core, is as much about our growth as it is about theirs. When you look back over the years, you begin to see not just the changes in your child, but in yourself. The man you are today has been shaped by sleepless nights, first-day-of-school nerves, difficult conversations, and moments of pure joy. Each experience has built a deeper well of empathy, patience, and wisdom.

Make time to honor that growth. Whether through journaling, quiet reflection, or heart-to-heart conversations with your partner or a trusted friend, take stock of who you are becoming. What have you learned about yourself as a father? What values have emerged as your compass? What are you most proud of, and what are you still working on?

You do not need to be a perfect dad. You only need to be a present one: a father who learns, adapts, and keeps showing up. Your willingness to keep growing is the greatest gift you can offer your child. It tells them that change is not something to fear, but something to embrace with courage and humility.

Evolving as a Father: Embracing Changing Roles

Adapting to the ever-changing landscape of parenting means recognizing when it's time to shift from being the hands-on guide your child once needed, to becoming a more observant, advisory presence as they grow older. This evolution calls for flexibility, patience, and the courage to let go of direct control while remaining a steady source of support and encouragement. It's essential to create an environment where children feel empowered to define their own aspirations and take active steps toward achieving them, knowing they have your guidance when needed.

Offering advice without dictating outcomes teaches them to trust their judgment, developing a deeper sense of accountability and independence. By resisting the urge to step in and fix every problem, you provide them with the space to encounter failure, discover resilience, and develop real-world problem-solving abilities.

Supporting your child's path to autonomy is not about stepping back entirely, it's about showing up differently, offering presence over interference. It involves recognizing that while they need the freedom to make their own choices, they still need to feel your consistent emotional availability and belief in their ability to navigate life. Establishing regular, open-hearted conversations can provide a bridge between their growing independence and your continued involvement.

These check-ins, casual or structured, offer opportunities to address concerns, celebrate wins, and deepen the emotional bond between you and your child. As your parenting style matures, so does your relationship, transitioning from one built on instruction to one rooted in mutual respect, shared trust, and emotional intimacy. Make it a habit to connect over more than rules and routines; talk about their aspirations, fears, friendships, and perspectives, ensure they always feel heard, validated, and understood.

Striking the right balance between independence and involvement is not a one-time achievement, it's an ongoing, dynamic process that requires your attention and growth. Each developmental stage your child enters will challenge you to reassess your role and find new ways to support their evolving needs and identity. Approach these changes with curiosity and grace, knowing that your willingness to evolve will not only strengthen your relationship but also equip your child to face the world with confidence and clarity.

Letting go doesn't mean stepping away, it means providing a strong, loving framework that encourages your child to stretch, grow, and thrive, with the knowledge that you'll always be there when it counts.

Reflecting on the Journey: Celebrating Your Growth as a Dad

As I sit surrounded by the presence of my children, I often find myself quietly reflecting on the long, humbling journey of fatherhood. These reflections are more than fond memories, they serve as mirrors of transformation, revealing how each experience has helped shape who I've become. Moments that once felt chaotic or overwhelming, those sleepless nights, moments of self-doubt, the balancing act between career and caregiving, now stand as markers of growth and resilience.

Through those challenges, I've found patience I didn't know I had and strength I never imagined I'd need.

Looking back helps me see not just how far my children have come, but how much I've grown right alongside them. Acknowledging that evolution reinforces my confidence as a father and prepares me to meet future challenges with a stronger, wiser heart. Engaging in reflective practice doesn't require grand gestures, it can begin with something as simple as keeping a journal.

Writing down your thoughts after a particularly tough day or recording a moment of unexpected joy can offer clarity and self-awareness that only hindsight brings. Over time, that journal becomes more than just a collection of entries, it becomes a living document of your parenting story, filled with lessons learned, victories celebrated, and growth witnessed.

Pair journaling with intentional self-check-ins and goal setting. Ask yourself regularly: Who am I as a father today? Who do I want to become tomorrow?

These mindful practices create a rhythm of continuous learning, pushing you to be more intentional, more present, and more loving in your role as a dad.
Celebrate the wins, big and small, with your family. These moments of joy and recognition build motivation, closeness, and a sense of shared purpose. Consider holding casual family reflections, perhaps during dinner or a walk, where everyone can talk about something they're proud of or something they've learned.

These conversations deepen emotional connection and offer a space where each family member's voice matters. Creating a scrapbook, memory box, or digital timeline of milestones and everyday moments also helps preserve these shared experiences in a tangible, meaningful way. Looking at those pictures, drawings, or notes serves as a visual affirmation of your family's growth and the love that has carried you through it all.

Reflecting on your parenting journey and celebrating how far you've come instills hope and purpose as you look ahead. With each phase, you gain new insight and tools to approach the next with renewed intention and strength. Use your reflections not as a final chapter, but as a launchpad for what's next, setting new goals, trying new strategies, and remaining open to growth.

Every stage of fatherhood, from infancy to adulthood, offers new chances to expand your capacity for love, patience, and wisdom. The small, quiet victories, being there when they need you, showing up with empathy, learning from your mistakes, are the ones that matter most in the long run. As you move forward, let your past experiences be both a teacher and a source of pride, reminding you of the incredible father you already are and the one you continue to become.

Conclusion: Looking Ahead with Confidence and Heart

As we come to the close of this journey, I hope you feel not only better prepared, but deeply empowered to enter this next chapter of fatherhood with strength and intention. We've unpacked what it means to be a present partner, an involved dad, and an emotionally aware caregiver navigating unfamiliar terrain.

At the core of this entire experience is emotional awareness, the ability to tune into not just your baby's needs, but also the emotional needs of your partner and yourself. The early stages of parenthood can feel overwhelming, but your presence, grounded, calm, and empathetic, is a powerful anchor that holds the family together.

Being present isn't simply about showing up; it's about engaging with openness and compassion in moments that matter most.

We also explored practical tools to help manage everyday challenges, from creating a sleep routine to understanding your baby's cues. These aren't just tricks; they're touchpoints that build connection, trust, and confidence in your evolving role.

Every diaper changed, every tear soothed, every moment of doubt navigated is part of building a foundation of love and trust. Your partnership with your co-parent remains a vital element of this journey. A healthy parenting partnership thrives on open communication, mutual respect, shared responsibilities, and unwavering support. You are not just co-parents, you are teammates setting an example for your child on what love, collaboration, and respect look like in action.

Equally vital is the sense of community you create around you. Whether it's with fellow dads, extended family, or online support groups, these connections remind you that you are never alone in this journey. Sharing your experience and hearing others' stories fosters camaraderie and offers wisdom that can't always be found in books. But know this: the journey doesn't end here. Fatherhood is a lifelong evolution. With every stage your child enters, you will be called to grow, stretch, and adapt again.

Keep seeking knowledge. Keep reflecting. Keep loving with intention. Remember, your role is powerful. The love, attention, and guidance you provide shape not only your child's life but the spirit of your entire family. Embrace this with a full heart, knowing that the moments you invest now leave an indelible legacy. Let each challenge be a steppingstone and each joy a reminder of what truly matters.

You have what it takes, and your family is better for having you in it.
You are enough.

You are growing.

You are deeply loved.

References

- *Dad Support Group - Postpartum Support International (PSI)* https://postpartum.net/group/dad-support-group/

- *New Dad Anxiety - How to Overcome the Fear of Fatherhood* https://www.daduniversity.com/blog/new-dad-anxiety-how-to-overcome-the-fear-of-fatherhood

- *The psychology behind being a dad and its effects on fathers ...* https://www.in-mind.org/article/the-psychology-behind-being-a-dad-and-its-effects-on-fathers-themselves#:~:text=Arguably%2C%20parenting%20is%20a%20major,the%20father%20identity%20%5B8%5D.

- *Redefining Fatherhood: A New Era of Masculinity in Today's World* https://www.poppylist.com/blog/redefining-fatherhood-a-new-era-of-masculinity-in-todays-world

- *Effects of Father-Neonate Skin-to-Skin Contact on Attachment* https://pmc.ncbi.nlm.nih.gov/articles/PMC5282438/#:~:text=New%20fathers%20have%20been%20shown,and%20enhance%20the%20dependency%20relationship.

- *Understanding Your Baby's Cues* https://texaswic.org/health-nutrition/baby/understanding-your-babys-cues

- *Baby's sleep routine: a father's role -
Naturalmat*
https://naturalmat.co.uk/blogs/news/baby-s-sleep-routine-a-father-s-role#:~:text=This%20is%20where%20dads%20can,and%20drowsy%2C%20ready%20for%20sleep.

- *Maximizing your paternity leave: A guide for new dads*
https://www.optimistdaily.com/2023/09/maximizing-your-paternity-leave-a-guide-for-new-dads/

- *Active Listening: The Super Power To Building Stronger ...* https://medium.com/dad-of-all-things/active-listening-the-super-power-to-building-stronger-bonds-with-your-kids-1f4caf41dd23

- *Validation in Relationships: The Importance of Emotional ...*
https://www.masterclass.com/articles/validation-in-relationships#:~:text=Getting%20validation%20from%20loved%20ones,can%20deepen%20your%20emotional%20connection.

- *How to fairly split chores and child care with a new baby at ...*
https://www.npr.org/2024/08/13/g-s1-14652/got-a-new-baby-how-to-fairly-split-chores-and-child-care-and-avoid-resentment

- *Postpartum depression - Symptoms and causes* https://www.mayoclinic.org/diseases-conditions/postpartum-depression/symptoms-causes/syc-20376617

- *Meal Prepping For New Dads: Set Yourself Up for Success* https://youate.com/tips/meal-prepping-for-new-dads-set-yourself-up-for-success/

- *Cleaning Schedule For Working Moms and Dads - Molly Maid* https://www.mollymaid.com/practically-spotless/cleaning-schedule-for-busy-parents/

- *Baby bath basics: A parent's guide* https://www.mayoclinic.org/healthy-lifestyle/infant-and-toddler-health/in-depth/healthy-baby/art-20044438

- *Family Routine: How to Create a Flexible Daily ...* https://justabasicmama.com/family-routine/

- *Help for Dads | Postpartum Support International (PSI)* https://www.postpartum.net/get-help/help-for-dads/

- *How to manage the stress of becoming a new dad* https://www.gidgetfoundation.org.au/fact-sheets/how-to-manage-the-stress-of-becoming-a-new-dad

- *Fatherhood group sessions: A descriptive and summative ...*

153

https://pmc.ncbi.nlm.nih.gov/articles/PMC7
756429/#:~:text=Fatherhood%20groups%20c
an%20help%20new,the%20space%20for%20s
uch%20discussions.

- *Self-care tips for expectant and new dads*
  https://www.gidgetfoundation.org.au/fact-
  sheets/self-care-tips-for-expectant-and-new-
  dads

- *Work-Life Balance – TOP 15 Tips for Working
  Parents* https://dad.ceo/article/faq-
  achieving-work-life-balance-for-busy-dads

- *THE IMPACT OF REMOTE WORK ON FAMILY
  DYNAMICS ...*
  https://papers.ssrn.com/sol3/Delivery.cfm/4
  856087.pdf?abstractid=4856087&mirid=1

- *Communicating Boundaries at Work*
  https://cerebral.com/care-
  resources/communicating-boundaries-at-
  work

- *The Benefits of Flexible Working for Parents*
  https://getofficely.com/blog/the-benefits-of-
  flexible-working-for-parents

- *Module 2: Understanding Children's
  Developmental Milestones*
  https://www.cdc.gov/ncbddd/watchmetrainin
  g/module2.html#:~:text=Looking%20for%20de
  velopmental%20milestones%20is,milestone%2
  0that%20signifies%20healthy%20development
  .

- *Tummy Time Tips*
  https://pathways.org/topics-of-development/tummy-time

- *Speech and Language Developmental Milestones*
  https://www.nidcd.nih.gov/health/speech-and-language

- *The Importance of Stimulating Environments for Children*
  https://www.philaymca.org/news/stimulating-environment-child-development

- *How To Deal With Sleep Deprivation After a Baby* https://www.parents.com/baby/new-parent/sleep-deprivation/how-to-get-sleep/

- *Colic - Diagnosis & treatment - Mayo Clinic*
  https://www.mayoclinic.org/diseases-conditions/colic/diagnosis-treatment/drc-20371081

- *Communicating with your partner in the perinatal period*
  https://www.panda.org.au/articles/communicating-with-your-partner-in-the-perinatal-period

- *Handling Unwanted Parenting Advice*
  https://app.mahmee.com/articles/handling-unwanted-parenting-advice

- *6 Tips on Being the Best Co-parenting Dad You Can Be* https://www.dcomply.com/6-tips-on-being-the-best-co-parenting-dad-you-can-be/

- *Conflict Resolution in Relationships & Couples: 5 Strategies* https://positivepsychology.com/conflict-resolution-relationships/

- *The Importance of Family Routines* https://www.healthychildren.org/English/fa mily-life/family-dynamics/Pages/The-Importance-of-Family-Routines.aspx

- *Parent Milestones Are Equally Important As Baby ...* https://www.businessinsider.com/parent-milestones-are-equally-important-as-baby-milestones-2023-6

- *Growth Mindset Parenting | Psychology Today* https://www.psychologytoday.com/us/blog/g oing-beyond-intelligence/202311/growth-mindset-parenting

- *Enhancing father involvement by increasing flexibility* https://journals.sagepub.com/doi/10.1177/1 3674935241295804?icid=int.sj-abstract.citing-articles.5

- *Perfecting Patience: Tips for Becoming a More Patient and ...* https://www.thefirmformen.com/articles/perf ecting-patience-tips-for-becoming-a-more-patient-and-understanding-father/

- *Postpartum Depression in Fathers: A Systematic Review*

https://pmc.ncbi.nlm.nih.gov/articles/PMC11122550/

- *Father Support Groups - A Guide to Support Groups for Dads* https://mensgroup.com/father-support-groups/

- *The Power of Storytelling* https://annemckeown.com/the-power-of-storytelling/

- *Fatherhood Mentoring & Unplanned Pregnancy Support* https://youhavealternatives.org/fatherhood-mentoring-program-application/

- *Why Family Traditions Are Important & How to Build Them* https://blog.nchs.org/why-are-family-traditions-important

- *6 Steps for Successful Family Goal Setting* https://spero.financial/6-steps-for-successful-family-goal-setting/

- *The Power of Positive Parenting | UC Davis Children Hospital* https://health.ucdavis.edu/children/patient-education/Positive-Parenting#:~:text=Neuroscientists%20discovered%20that%20positive%20parenting,cognition%20during%20the%20teen%20years.&text=Harvard%20scientists%20found%20that%20positive,and%20well%2Dbeing%20during%20adulthood.

- *Balancing Support and Independence to Promote Resilience* https://www.linkedin.com/pulse/balancing-emotional-validation-independence-promote-kids-buzanko-hyxbc#:~:text=Balancing%20emotional%20support%20with%20encouraging%20independence%20is%20a%20dynamic%20process,to%20navigate%20life's%20challenges%20successfully.

- *Reflective Practice: How Do You Really Feel about Fathers?* https://headstart.gov/family-engagement/father-engagement-strategies/reflective-practice-how-do-you-really-feel-about-fathers